EAT *Real* FOOD

Also by Julie Montagu

Books:

Superfoods: The Flexible Approach to Eating More Superfoods

DVDs:

21 Day Power Yoga, Detox and Weight Loss Method
with Julie Montagu

Online courses:

Nutrition for Optimal Health
(visit www.theflexifoodie.com for more information)

EAT *Real* FOOD

Simple Rules for Health, Happiness
and Unstoppable Energy

JULIE MONTAGU
THE FLEXI FOODIE

HAY HOUSE

Carlsbad, California • New York City • London • Sydney
Johannesburg • Vancouver • Hong Kong • New Delhi

Library of Congress Control Number: 2015959404

Tradepaper ISBN: 978-1-4019-4889-4

10 9 8 7 6 5 4 3 2 1
1st edition, April 2016

SUSTAINABLE FORESTRY INITIATIVE
Certified Chain of Custody
Promoting Sustainable Forestry
www.sfiprogram.org
SFI-01268
SFI label applies to the text stock

Printed in the United States of America

Allegra Whittome January 21,1999–February 7, 2015.
She exuded health, happiness, and unstoppable energy.

This book's for her: www.allegrasambition.org.uk

She needed a hero, so that's what she became.

Contents

Part I: My Simple Rules for Health

Learn how and why to include spinach, kale, Swiss chard, broccoli, and cabbage easily and effortlessly in your diet every day.

Learn how and why to include quinoa, millet, brown rice, oats, and buckwheat easily and effortlessly in your diet every day.

Learn how and why to include honey, brown rice syrup, maple syrup, date sugar, and coconut palm sugar or nectar easily and effortlessly in your diet every day.

Learn how and why to include olive oil, coconut oil, and flaxseed oil easily and effortlessly in your diet every day.

Part II: Simple Rules for Happiness and Unstoppable Energy

Acknowledgments

First and foremost, my husband Luke, who always believed in me even when I didn't! Thank you for being my personal cheerleader throughout this journey.

Emma, Jack, William and Nestor, my four superhero kids. Emma, thank you for sitting by my side on the sofa during the weekends while I wrote. You really kept me company and my spirits high. Jack, thank you for having so many rugby matches, which forced me to leave the writing for a bit, catch some much-needed fresh air, and root for you. William, your constant pats on the back and being so proud of your Mom, didn't go unnoticed. Thank you. And last but not least, Nestor. Thank you for cooking with me in the kitchen, tasting the recipes and even making some of your own, which truly inspired me, too.

Alix Jones, you are a miracle worker. For the past three years, you have been there to help me with so many last-minute requests and deadlines, and you've been such a huge asset while writing this book. Thank you.

Lucy Whittome, Allegra's Mom. I can't really put into words how much our friendship means to me. Thank you for always being so proud of me, even when times were tough, you lifted my spirits and I hope I can forever give that back to you.

Jonathan Sattin and Triyoga where for me it really all began. You've helped launch my career and I am forever grateful. One of the greatest things I've done is to teach yoga and to be able to teach at Triyoga… well, for me, it doesn't get any better than that.

Sandy Draper for seriously perfecting this book. Your comments, notes, edits have helped make this book better than I ever imagined. Thank you.

Amy Kiberd and Ruth Tewkesbury at Hay House—from the first meeting at Dayleford to now. I still pinch myself that this book is here and it's all thanks to you, your belief in me, and your amazing, continued support. Thank you.

Thank you to everyone at Hay House UK and USA. Having this book published by you is simply a dream come true.

And last, thank you to YOU. All of you out there who have believed in me, supported me, and sent me the most wonderfully kind messages. I wouldn't be where I am today if it weren't for your constant words of encouragement and positivity. This book is for you.

How to Make "Simple" Work

"Eat food, not too much, mostly plants."
MICHAEL POLLAN

I love the definition of simple: Easy to understand, not elaborate, or complicated. Not complex... But what's happened to the 'simple' in eating and in our diet? When did it all become so overcomplicated? There are now thousands of diet books to choose from—but do they work, *really*? Or do they just make eating more difficult? Who, what, and which diet is right for you in the end?

We all know deep down that diets simply don't work. I feel as if the word diet has somehow morphed into a new definition of achieving a goal in an unrealistically short amount of time, during which we feel awful and even filled with resentment, depression, and guilt.

Why can't we just eat as they did back in the golden olden days when calories weren't counted or didn't even matter! Our ancestors ate to live—they needed energy to sustain themselves to gather fruits, vegetables, legumes, nuts and seeds, and for hunting meat. They used up their food supplies quickly because there weren't any chemicals or refrigerators to make them last longer. They didn't have to read labels or count calories because they consumed whole foods that gave them the necessary energy and nutritional benefits they needed to survive and thrive. Their diet included salt, fats, and sugars, which they consumed in their whole states with nothing artificially added in.

Think about how eating a home-cooked meal of whole foods is satisfying, filling, and nutrient rich. Now think back to a time when you consumed a commercially, ready-made, processed, packaged meal. How did it make you feel? Most likely lethargic and, perhaps, not very satisfied. That's because these processed options are stripped of nutrients and filled with empty calories. Mother Nature is smarter than any processed food company out there. Think about it… we are attracted to brightly colored, whole foods from juicy red apples to dark green spinach. But it seems to me that many food manufacturers are trying to become their own Mother Nature by deceiving us. They want to trick us into believing that these manufactured foods are good for us because they have been brightened with colors and enhanced with 'fake' flavors.

My view is that we started getting sicker and fatter when we began consuming and counting calories that came from anything and everything but real, whole foods. Who has the time to count calories anyway? Isn't that just one more thing to add to our long lists of "to do" each and every day? I sometimes laugh about what my ancestors would think if they saw me microwave a plastic container filled with some sort of good-for-me meal. A meal that has been made in a factory, pumped with chemicals and preservatives so that it can last longer in my refrigerator. Then, after consuming it, I write the calories consumed in my booklet that accompanies the two weeks' worth of packaged "diet" foods I'd bought…

I tell my clients to make sure they recognize every single listed ingredient on the labels of packaged foods—and there should never be more than five or six. For example, let's consider cereal. I would much rather eat granola made from whole seeds, nuts, and grains than something filled with ingredients that I've never even heard of before.

So, the burning question is: Can we really go back to "simple" and will we then feel better, have more energy, lose weight, lower our cholesterol, still enjoy our food, and be happy?

The short answer is a big, fat yes! I want to show you what I have been doing for the past eight years, ever since my youngest child was born. This way of living has not only worked for me but at the ripe age of 40 (something) and four kids later, I now feel the best I have felt in years. My energy rocks a whole new level and my health has never been better, a.k.a. lovely blood pressure, perfect resting heart rate, and low cholesterol, to name just a few. This is all due to adding in the good stuff—food, breathing, yoga, meditation, and affirmations—that naturally crowd out the bad stuff. Trust me.

How do I make "simple" work?

Let's remember the facts first. I think we all know that when we eat less saturated fat, less cholesterol, and more fiber, we help our bodies with "disease prevention." Do you know which foods contain no bad saturated fat or cholesterol and have loads of fiber, phytonutrients, and antioxidants? Yup, wholesome plant-based foods. But it can be complicated when you go shopping for food, right? There are aisles of processed and packaged foods everywhere. It seems to me that grains, veggies, and fruits are always hidden away in the periphery of the grocery store. This is kind of sad in my view! But starting right now, right here, we have the power to change that. To change our shopping and eating habits, and in return get real, authentic energy, glowing skin, happy moods, and the power to prevent and even heal from illnesses.

I love-love-love the quote from the inspirational Michael Pollan, a nutritionist and bestselling author of *In Defense of Food*, who says "Eat food. Not too much. Mostly plants." So if you are wondering whether you should go, vegetarian, paleo, vegan, or even raw, then ask yourself, "Shouldn't I just do what my ancestors did and keep things simple?"

The simpler we keep things, the easier it is to wade through the crazy amount of information that's out there on "what diet to try next." So my main aim in this book is to show how simple always works best. And while we're on the subject of "diets," when I refer to the word "diet" in this book, I am talking about what we are meant to be eating those whole foods, not the processed ones. Trust me, once you say goodbye to a diet packed with processed, packaged "junk" food and hello to a yummy, plant-fuelled diet comprised of mostly veggies, fruits, grains, nuts, seeds, and natural sweeteners, your taste buds will change and any excess weight will simply glide off with little effort. You'll start to look forward to new recipes, new whole-food discoveries, and a whole new you—which in turn will bring you to gleaming health, bounding with energy, and feeling heaps of happiness.

The start of a simple journey

The "Simple Rules", as I call them, are the ones that I've been living by for a while now, and personally I've found that they've made making healthy choices so much easier. However, I've found that the key to success comes in really understanding *why* the healthy food choices *are* healthy, and knowing all of the amazing things that these foods can do for the body. When you know what the benefits are you won't want to go without them. Although it may seem like a lot of information to take in at first, if you adapt your life slowly to incorporate one rule at a time, then you soon won't even notice that you are following them! So here follows the Simple

Rules in a nutshell and start on our simple journey toward eating a healthy, nutritious diet.

Eat wholesome, plant-based foods

First of all, flood your kitchen with wholesome, plant-based foods. If it is processed or comes in a packet with a long list of ingredients on the label then the chances are it is not good for you. When you do this, you will immediately notice that your refrigerator and your cupboards are filled with so much more color. Stop buying the foods that don't fit into the concept of simple and focus on plant-based and whole-grain varieties. Think of it as your mission to incorporate more good foods into your kitchen because having some whole foods in your diet is better than none. Then think of me as your cheerleader, to cheer you on, to share more ideas, to create more interesting recipes that can help you get to the top of the pyramid and shout to those in the bleachers, "I feel amazing!"

But more than tasting great and being super fun to cook with, whole foods contain the fiber we need to keep our systems moving. They are packed full of the natural antioxidants that our bodies crave to fight free radicals, and crammed with phytonutrients to protect us from disease. Let's zoom in quickly on the three key things that whole foods give us in abundance.

1. Fiber

This keeps things moving through the digestive system and out of the body, but it also contains other benefits, such as lowering our risk of diabetes, keeping our hearts healthy, and even preventing certain cancers.

2. Phytonutrients

These make the carrots orange, the blueberries blue, and that kale super green but also protect the plants against disease, enemies, UV rays, and environmental pollutants to name just a few. And, these fighters—a.k.a. phytonutrients—can do the same for our bodies.

3. Antioxidants

We hear the word antioxidants everywhere nowadays. This is high in antioxidants and so is that and so is that, but that one is not, etc. But do we really know what an antioxidant is and why they are good for us?

Antioxidants are found in many whole foods and these nutrients can protect us against free radicals. Free radical lesson 101 teaches us that these guys can damage our cells and be the foundations for disease. The problem is we can't stop free radicals from forming because they are constantly reacting with oxygen, which in turn we need to stay alive.

A good way to understand how free radicals can affect our health is by thinking about what happens when we peel and chop a banana. After being exposed to the air, the banana turns brown— that's the oxidation process in real live action. Those brown parts are the free radicals forming and it is impossible to avoid these puppies. In the same way, the human body is also exposed to oxygen and so free radicals are forming in us all of the time—whether from breathing in exhaust fumes from the traffic we sit in or from working out, or even from digesting our food. But we can combat these guys by consuming antioxidants in the foods we eat every single day. Antioxidants are our protectors, they are our superheroes, and we want to get as many of them into our bodies as possible to block the damage that free radicals can cause.

Literally, the food we eat makes all the difference, and not some "magic" pill.

Listen to your body

Which leads me on to my next "keep it simple" tip—it's called listening to your body. Really listening. When the body gets sick that's its way of crying out for help. However, because it can't tell us in words, the body shows us in the form of a cold, a headache, a rash, a bad mood, some cramps, and even constipation. Most of us have been conditioned to think that popping a pill will cure a lot of these bodily cries for help, whereas, most of the time, medications often cause more symptoms in the form of side effects. Meds mask the cold, the cramping, the congestion, the constipation, and the moods. If we develop a rash or some skin irritability, it is likely that our body is trying to get rid of toxins by pushing them out through the skin. Or if we are having a hard time eliminating them, it is most likely that our bodies are not getting what they need—fiber.

Think of your body like a car for a second. What happens if you give your car diesel when it needs unleaded? It breaks down, of course! The same applies to our bodies. If we are not feeding them the right fuel, they are going to break down. But have no fear because we can repair our bodies with what we put in our mouths—whole foods. The cries out from our bodies—a.k.a. the symptoms—are almost always evidence of something bigger that we can treat by changing our eating habits and lifestyles. But sadly, popping a pill is easier and takes a lot less effort than changing our habits. So the first pill (no pun intended) to swallow is forward planning.

Yes, at first some forward planning will be required in order to create meals and snacks that consist of whole, healthy foods, which will also mean learning how to create more space for you. But you will soon find you easily adapt to this new, simpler way of eating and living. Before you know it, these changes will have become healthy habits because whole foods truly give us the opportunity to have fun in the kitchen, explore new recipes, and discover interesting ingredients. Personally, I think making a Quinoa and Red Pepper Chili (*see page 51 for the recipe*) makes for a much more fun and interesting meal than a pan-fried steak plopped alongside some boiled carrots and mashed potatoes. Additionally, even taking just five minutes out of your day for some breathing or meditation, or even a forward fold, gives that little bit of energy and happiness back to yourself.

Eat an energizing breakfast

The old mantra that breakfast is the most important meal of the day continues to ring true. I know a lot of us have become so busy with life that we have gotten into the habit of slugging a coffee and maybe consuming a sugar-laced muffin, a cereal bar, or a refined flour bagel. Or, to sum it up, a bunch of empty calories that are stripped of nutrients. Think of breakfast as setting the tone for the rest of your day—I am serious about that! Trust me, you simply will not lose weight by skipping breakfast. You will, however, screw up your metabolism and possibly even become a morning grump. When I am hungry, I am grumpy!

Breakfast means "breaking" the "fast." You wake up in the morning and haven't eaten since the night before, so it has likely been 10 hours since your last meal. That is a good thing as it gives your body time to rest, digest, and reset. But when we wake up in the morning we are moving again and we are thinking again, therefore we need to be on top form. By eating breakfast you are waking up your metabolism and getting it revved-up for the day. Eating breakfast wakes up your brain, making you more alert and ready to take on the world. If you start out with a healthy breakfast of whole foods then you are more likely to choose something healthy for lunch, too. It is all about starting the day on the right foot by engaging right away with your health and wellness. It takes time to change unhealthy habits so making a habit of a healthy breakfast every morning is a great way to start the change.

Remember, adding in the good stuff will eventually overtake the bad stuff, so just take your time and enjoy this adventure every step of the way. With an energizing breakfast you will be nutritionally equipped for the day ahead. Also, with your morning meal, it is important to have a good balance of protein, beneficial fats, and carbohydrates.

Grains are a good high protein choice for breakfast, especially oats or quinoa, both of which can be used to make a nutrient-dense porridge. Good fat sources such as avocado or nuts go well as a breakfast accompaniment too, and healthy carbohydrates can be acquired from a wide range of fruits, vegetables, and whole grains.

> With the right breakfast, you will have all of the energy you need to get through until lunchtime, and without reaching for a sugary snack or caffeinated drink.

Check out some of my breakfast recipes *(see pages 54, 56, 85, and 125)* to find out how to kick-start your day with foods that will nourish and energize you for the day ahead.

Concentrate on whole foods first

A whole food is defined as a food that has been processed or refined as little as possible, and is free from additives or other artificial substances. Even though the content and recipes in this book do not include any animal products or processed and packaged foods, *Eat Real Food* is not about deprivation. In fact, the opposite is true!

Once you have the facts and the tools to easily incorporate a large variety of whole foods into your diet, you'll soon realize the amazing benefits of doing so in all of your daily meals. Once I went back to basics and got rid of the complicated, I found that I had more energy to exercise, to cycle to my yoga classes every day, to teach my yoga classes, and also to be a happier mother, wife, and friend. I had a clearer headspace so I was able to do more. In a nutshell, since turning to a whole-food diet, I have never felt better—ever.

The advantage of whole foods is that they're packed full of fiber, as well as vitamins and minerals, which is often lost in processed or refined foods.

By incorporating whole foods into your diet, you'll be providing your body with a huge boost of nutrition that it is starved of with processed foods. This in itself will give your energy levels a noticeable lift. Whole foods protect your body against health problems and promote life-long health. I am, of course, talking about greens, fruits, whole grains, beans, legumes, water, nuts, seeds, unrefined oil, natural sweeteners, and superfoods—the aim is to get these good guys in every single day!

Refuel with priority proteins

When you cut back on the meat and add in more whole foods, you are getting the fiber, beta-carotene, vitamin C, vitamin K, folic acid, magnesium, and potassium into your diet while cutting right back on the saturated fat and cholesterol. However, since meat-free diets became popular people have been quick to doubt their nutritious value due to the inability to provide a complete protein. This logic is clearly flawed but allow me to explain why.

There are 20 different amino acids and these are the essential building blocks of protein. The body is able to produce 11 of these amino acids by itself and the other nine are taken from the foods we eat—they are known as essential amino acids. Although plant-based foods do not contain complete proteins, they do provide a wide range of different essential amino acids. This means that by eating a varied, plant-based diet, you can easily hit your necessary amino acid quota and therefore your protein quota. The great thing about plant-based proteins is that we can get them from a whole host of sources, such as quinoa, legumes, nuts, seeds, lentils, buckwheat, and even rice.

If you make sure that you consume a high protein food with each meal, such as quinoa, buckwheat, chia seeds, or rice and beans, then your body will continue to refuel throughout the day.

> Include a variety of grains, legumes, fruit and vegetables in your daily diet, and you'll get all the protein you need.

Experiment with superfoods

Some foods branded with the superfood label have been questioned over the years, as cynics put this term down to marketing hype. However, it has to be noted that there is much indisputable evidence that a selection of foods provide a much higher nutrient count than others. So let's get down to business. It is becoming clearer and clearer that superfoods are both food *and* medicine due to being packed with super-potent, super-concentrated nutrients. They are fantastic for meeting, and even exceeding, all of our amino acids, vitamins, minerals, and essential fatty acids requirements, and have been shown to provide more bang for your buck. In other words, more nutrition with less eating! I always try to eat at least one superfood every single day, whether that's soaked chia seeds for breakfast, a cacao smoothie, or a goji berry energy ball. Think of superfoods as your fountain of youth, health, and wellness.

Choosing to include these foods in your diet can bring a wide range of benefits, such as bolstering your immune system, cleansing your body, and improving your overall health. It also brings some diversity to mealtimes. The Simple Rules will help guide you to choosing different superfoods and make it simple to include them in your everyday meals.

Do one activity a day just for you

Taking time for you is extremely underrated, but is important in order to maintain a sense of freedom, control, and general wellbeing. If you are constantly rushing from one task to the next due to a stressful or demanding job or taking care of a family or both, then you are going to burn out quickly!

Setting aside a little time for you can help you to unwind from the pressures of the day and restore some peace in your mind. This should be a fraction of the day where you can be completely alone with no interruptions or distractions. Switch off your phone, move away from the computer, and make sure nobody is going to disturb. You may find this hard to do at first, particularly if you're used to being completely consumed by your demanding schedule, but you will soon see the benefits.

> Even if it is just five minutes a day, find the
> opportunity to schedule some me time.

A few great ways to use this time are to do some breathing exercises, meditation, drink a green juice, say some wonderful affirmations, or even do a couple of yoga poses... whatever you do, it will be just for you! When we give back to ourselves, we are more equipped and more able to give back to those we love, and, more importantly, the more we will start to love ourselves. The more you nourish you from the inside out, the more energy and happiness you will cultivate.

The benefits of the "Simple Rules"

There is no diet on the planet that will cure every ailment and combat all of the negative factors associated with aging. However, following my Simple Rules will equip your body with the ability to better prevent and fight disease, as well as refreshing your skin, boosting your energy levels, and helping to promote optimum brain function—all of which will leave you feeling and looking younger!

Protect your body

There is now overwhelming evidence that shows eating more whole foods significantly affects our state of health. We are NOT meant to have inflammation, high blood sugar, high blood pressure, high cholesterol, or aches and pains. Eating whole foods does much more than fill our bellies. They can help prevent and even treat disease and illness. Whole foods can affect how we feel, how we look, how much we weigh, how we age, and how much energy we have. So let's eat for pleasure because we need to have some fun in life and eating is definitely a source of fun. Let's combine that with a diet that protects us, heals us, and makes us feel great every single day.

Clear your head

Finding the time to include yoga in your day will help you feel relaxed and manage your stress levels, while also improving your stamina, flexibility, strength, and much more. Absolutely anyone can participate in, and benefit from, some form of yoga, so just let go of whatever is holding you back. You can choose to learn by taking classes or even in your own living room using one of the huge selection of instructional videos available online.

Meditation and breathing exercises often go hand in hand, but that doesn't mean you can't use them separately. Meditation can be achieved with just a few moments of peace and focus, as can a breathing exercise. Both of these simple practices promote a sense of calm while also helping you to become more present. It is effortless to get started with meditation, as it also is with breathing exercises. Both of these activities can quickly bring immense benefits to your mental health and wellbeing

Affirmations are a fantastic way to bring a quick dose of positivity and motivation into any moment. The great thing about affirmations is that you can do them anytime, anywhere, and they only take a few moments! They will help to eradicate negative thoughts from your mind and to remind you of all the great things about your life and being you.

You'll find more on yoga, meditation, breathing, and affirmations in Chapter 8, when we'll look at the many benefits of all four practices in more detail, and you'll find some exercises to set you on the path to feeling calmer, more energized, and more flexible.

Lower blood pressure

Vegetarian and vegan diets have long been associated with lower blood pressure and several studies[1] have confirmed this. Although my Simple Rules don't necessarily require you to eradicate meat, fish, or animal products entirely, I would encourage you to substantially increase your consumption of plant-based and natural whole foods.

Normal blood pressure is less than 120/80mmHg and high blood pressure is one of the biggest threats to our precious, beating hearts. One of the main ways to control your blood pressure is to keep the amount of salt you eat to a minimum, but that can be hard to do on a diet rich in processed and packaged foods—which are usually laden with added salt. But, by following the advice in this book, you'll be adding more whole foods to your diet and so looking after your blood pressure and your heart. Eating this way, you may also find that any excess weight drops off naturally and being a healthy weight is one of the best ways of maintaining a healthy blood pressure. Excess body weight is linked to high blood pressure and those who follow a plant-based diet are much more likely to weigh less than those who don't.

The reason that a plant-based diet protects your hearts is that as we decrease the amount of animal fats and increase the amount of whole foods, we naturally start eating cleaner, simpler foods. In turn, your blood becomes cleaner and the heart doesn't have to push as hard to move the blood around your body. These whole foods are low in the saturated fats that are found in meats and dairy, so your blood pressure naturally returns to a healthier level. In fact, studies have shown that plant-based diets lower blood pressure rather quickly.[2] As an extra bonus, fruits and veg are loaded with potassium, and this also helps to regulate blood pressure, as well as protecting mental wellbeing, and defending the body against the negative effects of stress.

By choosing to participate regularly in yoga, meditation, and/or breathing exercises, you will also be protecting your heart because relaxation reduces blood pressure. So not only will your body be calmer and less stressed during these practices, but you will also equip your mind with the ability to remain in a more relaxed state throughout the day. As a result, you may find it easier to approach difficult situations and less prone to panic about the small things that used to make you feel stressed.

Lower blood cholesterol

Bad cholesterol, also known as "LDL cholesterol," is commonly known to be a factor in heart disease and strokes because it increases the risk of blockages in the arteries. Plant-based, whole foods not only lower LDL cholesterol levels but also protect against poor health conditions that arise due to high cholesterol. The problem is we can usually see the fat in animal products, but we can't see the cholesterol. And here's the shocker—most of the cholesterol from animal products often hides in the lean parts! But plants are different. Veggies, fruits, and other plant foods contain zero cholesterol. Yup, that's right! I said zero cholesterol, and so this simple change in your diet can have a huge impact on your blood cholesterol level. There are countless examples of people decreasing, or indeed stopping, their consumption of animal-based products and increasing the amounts of plant-based whole foods. The result of which is that their bad cholesterol levels significantly decrease.

Better blood sugar

The consumption of sugary convenience, processed, and packaged foods can be seen to have increased in line with the rising incidence of type 2 diabetes in recent years. When it comes to blood sugar, insulin is the prime component to consider, as it tells the body to absorb glucose from the blood system. Glucose, the sugar in our blood, is the main fuel for the body. The problem arises when glucose can't get into the cells of our body where it needs to be. Instead it travels around the blood in our bodies at freakishly high levels. Diabetes also increases the risk of damage to the heart and blood vessels. On average, people with type 2 diabetes, who don't manage the disease well, risk losing about a decade of life compared to those who don't have the disease. What a shame!

By following my Simple Rules, you'll be swapping refined sugar for natural, whole food alternatives. Refined sugars are a leading cause of glucose problems as the body not only breaks them down incredibly quickly but they have also been stripped of all their nutrients. Natural alternatives are slow releasing, have lots of health benefits, are packed with nutrients, and have good levels of fiber. Eating these foods therefore leads to more balanced blood sugar levels, and so creates a healthier you.

Lower rates of cancer

As we discussed earlier (*see page xvii*), whole foods contain potent phytonutrients to combat and fight off the negative effects of free radicals, which can lead to cancer. Remember, phytonutrients are naturally occurring in plants and help to protect the plants from disease and more. These same phytonutrients, when consumed by us, work with our bodies to help fight cancer by keeping the cells reproducing normally and so preventing cell mutation. Research has long shown that a diet rich in foods with high counts of antioxidants helps to keep diseases, and especially cancer, at bay.[3] My Simple Rules encourage you to seek color in your produce because dark green, orange, red, yellow, and purple plant-based foods are known to have an especially high phytonutrient count. The Simple Rules also suggest that you include plenty of cruciferous vegetables and citrus fruits, which contain especially high numbers of disease-fighting phytochemicals, too.

Weight loss

What if you could speed up your metabolism and convert what you eat into energy rather than store it as fat? Now wouldn't that be nice? Most people think that one of the only ways to speed up the metabolism is to exercise—and exercise a lot. But did you know that you could also speed up your metabolism, which of course aids weight loss, by simply adding more whole foods to your diet? Our metabolism helps us turn fuel into energy but if we don't eat the right stuff, then some of that fuel is redundant and so stored as fat. The body needs fuel to run and therefore to burn, so the faster your metabolism, the faster you will burn calories and the less you will store fat.

So how can we speed up our metabolism? Simple. Every time we eat a meal rich in plant-based whole foods, nutrients pass into the bloodstream and then on to and into the cells of our body, where they are converted to energy or fuel for the body. Just like throwing wood on a fire, our metabolism speeds up when we give it the right foods. And, as a bonus, consuming a diet high in whole foods means our metabolism stays a bit higher for a few hours after eating. So it is literally a win–win situation. Plant-based whole foods are the essence of the Simple Rules and those who follow a plant-based diet generally have a lower BMI (body mass index; to calculate your BMI visit www.smartbmicalculator.com) than omnivores. Making gradual changes to eradicate processed, high-sugar foods in favor of natural alternatives, you'll likely see a progressive and permanent reduction in your weight and a boost to your overall health.

Increased energy

Processed foods and animal products are generally quite difficult to digest, meaning your body has to use a lot of energy to get the job done. Digestion sucks our energy because it uses a lot more energy than most of the other processes in the body. So if we consume foods that our bodies can't use—due to being laden with additives, preservatives, too much added sugar, salt, and fat—then our energy levels drop because our body needs more energy to digest them. This is why a diet abundant in these foods will leave you feeling drained and perpetually tired.

> Simple wholesome foods are not only high in energy-inducing nutrients but are also easy to digest, so won't tax your energy levels. This in turn will help you to bounce through each and every day.

Practicing yoga, breathing exercises, and meditation is also great for our energy levels because these calming activities help us to reset and refresh. By engaging in them every day, we allow our bodies time to recharge in a positive and natural way. When our energy is low, sometimes all we need is to take time out to get back on track. Doing a few simple yoga poses, peaceful meditation, or mindful breathing exercises encourages our mind to relax as our energy levels zoom back up.

Longer life span

Obviously a diet rich in plant-based whole foods doesn't mean we are going to live forever but it can add years to our lives. Rather than being struck down by illness, extra weight, and low energy, we can really live during the time we have and enjoy this thing called life to the full.

Regular yoga practice can also help to promote optimum health and this also leads to a longer life span. This is not only due to the physical benefits of yoga but also because it teaches us to deal with stress, which can be a serious detriment to our health! Meditation and breathing exercises also give us stress-coping mechanisms by encouraging us to slow down and contemplate the things that are really important in life, leading us to worry less about the insignificant things.

Simple tips on making the change

Carving out a time each week to create your meal plan for the week ahead is a rather fun thing to do. Pick a slot in your diary each week, so that it is there, and then spend a couple of hours finding and working on recipes, ideas, and shopping lists.

You might also want to dedicate another slot during the week to going shopping for the items on your shopping list. When you return home, store your produce, veggies, etc., and soak your nuts, seeds, and grains, if needed. Take this time to then prepare any dressings and sauces in advance. You can chop up the vegetables or other ingredients that you will be using over the next couple of days and freeze them. You can even squeeze all of your lemons and keep the juice in an airtight container in the fridge for up to two weeks.

If you know you are going to have a tough week ahead then make a few dishes in advance and freeze them for the upcoming week. Many of the recipes in this book make large batches so you can make several portions at a time and pop them in the freezer for when you need to rustle up a quick meal.

Find a friend to join forces with and do your shopping together and then share your recipes and meal ideas for the week ahead. This not only encourages you to stick to your schedule, but can also inspire you to seek out new ideas to share with friends. You will also have the benefit of having their ideas shared with you!

> If you have leftovers from dinners, then either freeze them for another night's dinner or use them the next day for lunch. This saves you having to cook the following day and makes sure that none of your delicious, nutrient-packed food or hard work goes to waste!

Leave room for creativity and improvisation. Sometimes we don't have time for a plan and that is OK. Believe me, it happens to me! So when you're in a bind and super busy, remember that all recipes don't need to be followed to a "T"—and you can use whatever you have to hand. For example, if you don't have kale, use spinach. No quinoa, use brown rice. No cashews then use another nut. No dried cranberries, use raisins. No maple syrup, use honey. You get the gist.

It is also important to set aside a designated time for your yoga, meditation, and breathing exercises. Even though they are all useful tools for immediate relief from a stressful situation and therefore may be utilized during the day, it also helps to have a scheduled time and space for more intense and deliberate practice.

You may find it most useful to do these things in the morning to prepare yourself for the day ahead or alternatively in the evening to allow yourself time to unwind and de-stress. Whichever option works best for you is fine as long as you focus solely on the task at hand with no distractions. If this means you have to set your alarm 10 minutes earlier in the morning or switch off 10 minutes sooner in the evening then make the sacrifice! Find a comfortable area that promotes relaxation and turn it into your sanctuary for peace. This will soon become a place and time that you look forward to during your day.

The start of your simple journey to a healthier you

The power to change and create new healthier habits takes time so don't beat yourself up if these changes don't happen overnight. They shouldn't. It is called taking baby steps for a reason! When we go out of our "norm" and start to try to break old habits, in order to create new ones, it always takes time. We all have insecurities when it comes to trying something new. We ask ourselves, "What if I don't have all the right ingredients for this recipe?" "I don't think my family is going to come on board with me," "Will my friends laugh at me?" "What if I mess up?"

I always tell my kids that if we didn't fail from time to time then we wouldn't appreciate what winning feels like—it would be boring—we would be boring. Going into the unknown can be scary, but that is also where amazing things are waiting for us. Take it slow and keep it simple. Start by changing one habit then move on to the next and the next and so on and so on. Change doesn't happen overnight. It is not instantaneous. It takes time, commitment, and few mistakes along the way. But I promise you it is worth it!

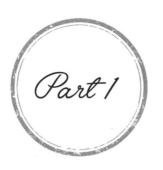

Part 1

My Simple Rules for Health

I like to think of Part I of this book as, what I call, the "Flexi-Five." We've been told for years and years and years that we need to get more fruits and veg into our diets by eating "five a day." Well, the Flexi-Five is a similarly simple philosophy and perhaps even more powerful, so just remember: Get one green leafy veg in a day as well as one whole grain, one natural sweetener, one healthy fat or oil, and one superfood, and you're on a seriously simple journey to better health!

Chapter 1

Eat One Green Leafy Veg Every Day

Learn how and why to include spinach, kale, Swiss chard, broccoli, and cabbage easily and effortlessly in your diet every day.

Believe it or not, green leafy vegetables are the most omitted food in our modern-day diet. Kinda shocking, right? It is even more shocking when we consider the wealth of goodness that these vegetables contain. Green vegetables are an amazing source of minerals, most notably magnesium, potassium, calcium, and iron. Add to that they contain high numbers of vitamins such as vitamin A, C, E, K, and a variety of the all-important B vitamins. These vitamins and minerals are all incredibly important for optimum health and, although it is possible to get them from other sources, eating green vegetables provides a way to get an abundance of them in the same place in relatively small servings.

With such a choice of green vegetables available, there is also a massive range of textures and flavors—so there is bound to be something for everyone. Understanding the amazing benefits that these vegetables have is a great way to motivate ourselves to include them in our diet. Even more so when we truly realize how simple it can be.

Greens help to purify the blood

The effectiveness of the blood-circulation system has an impact on the health of the rest of our bodies and, for that reason, it is super essential and super important that we not only take care of it but also make it a priority. Here follows a little lesson 101 on how our blood works.

The blood carries oxygen and nutrients around the body, and carries carbon dioxide away from the cells, ensuring optimum function. The kidneys and liver are tasked with keeping the blood free of toxins. If the blood isn't able to deliver oxygen and nutrients to the kidneys and the liver, then their functions quickly become impaired and this can rapidly lead to much bigger problems in the form of health issues.

The inclusion of green vegetables in your diet also helps your body to neutralize chemicals that have been ingested during mealtimes. Unless you eat organic 100 percent of the time then you are going to be consuming pesticides and even small amounts of certain metals when you eat. It is important that the good outweighs the bad when considering this and green veg are an effective weapon. They are your best friends when it comes to enemies in the body.

And last, by providing your body with the right foods, a.k.a. these dark green leafy vegetables, you can assist the blood in removing toxins from your system. Green vegetables are known to be a rich source of essential nutrients, making them beneficial for purifying the blood. The high antioxidant count of green vegetables makes them a strong tool for the liver to use in detoxifying and keeping the blood clean. This in turn means that your body remains clean and healthy, too. Think about it... the cleaner the blood, the happier the body.

How greens can protect us from cancer

Cancer starts when certain cells within the body begin to divide out of control. This mutation can occur for a number of reasons but it is commonly due to the presence of carcinogens in the body. It is, of course, impossible to protect ourselves from carcinogens completely, but what we can do is protect our cells through proper nutrition. When our body is properly equipped to defend itself, the occurrence of mutations and other diseases becomes lower. One of the best weapons that we can obtain from food for cancer prevention is carotenoids.[1]

Dark leafy green vegetables, such as kale, spinach, Swiss chard, chicory, and mustard greens are a particularly good source of lutein and zeaxanthin—both types of carotenoids. As the human body is incapable of producing carotenoids, it is essential to obtain them through the foods we eat and there are approximately 600 different types. When they enter the body, carotenoids act as antioxidants, helping to protect the body against cellular damage. Within carotenoids are acetylenic metabolites that are proven to work against the development of tumors and harmful organisms that may present themselves in the body.

Research into the effectiveness of carotenoids in cancer prevention has shown that they work by seeking out free radicals before they have a chance to cause any damage.[2] Although it would be wrong to say that this prevents all cancers, there is already strong evidence to show that cancers of the mouth are much less prevalent when there is a strong presence of carotenoids. Further research has also shown carotenoids are useful in inhibiting cancerous growths of the skin, breasts, lungs, and stomach.[3,4]

Green vegetables are crammed full of other nutrients and antioxidants that are also known to help in cancer prevention.[5] The majority of vegetables in this group contain high levels of a group of substances called glucosinolates—natural chemicals that contain sulfur. They are mostly responsible for the flavor and smell of green vegetables.

When these glucosinolates are broken down during digestion, they produce a range of compounds and these are currently being studied for their anti-cancer properties. It is believed that they not only protect cells from damage but also that they are capable of deactivating carcinogens.[6,7]

> Greens are great for general health as they have anti-inflammatory, antiviral, and antibacterial properties.

So far this research suggests that prostate cancer, colorectal cancer, lung cancer, and breast cancer are inhibited most by a high consumption of the glucosinolates in green vegetables.[8-11]

Greens improve circulation

Every cell in your body relies on oxygen in order to function properly, which means that your circulatory system has an incredibly important job to do. The circulatory system comprises of your heart and many thousands of miles of blood vessels! As well as delivering oxygen, the circulatory system also carries hormones and nutrients to the cells, and moves toxins to the kidneys so that they can be safely expelled from the body.

Green vegetables, and in particular dark, leafy green vegetables, are high in iron, which is essential for making red blood cells—the cells responsible for circulating oxygen through the system. It is thought that men and women need different amounts of iron in their diets but that we should all aim for 8–18mg per day.

However, if you are a pregnant then you may need to eat more and increase your iron intake to closer to 30mg per day.

Green vegetables are also high in vitamin E and so can improve circulation, as well as keeping the blood vessels flexible and open. With a vitamin E deficiency the potential for a narrowing of the arteries exists. By keeping your blood vessels in optimum shape, you are helping to protect yourself against cardiovascular disease.

Vitamin C, which is also plentiful in green vegetables, works to keep your blood vessels healthy, too. Vitamin C is especially useful for producing the collagen that holds tissue together. If your vitamin C levels are low then you are at risk of weak blood vessels that can eventually rupture and prevent circulation to the affected area.

Greens strengthen the immune system

The majority of the immune system is focused in the gut so if your gut is unhealthy then your immune system is going to suffer, too. It has been discovered that a fully functional immune system relies on a gene known as T-bet. This gene is essential for producing immune cells in the gut and it is now understood that it specifically responds to green vegetables.[12]

Many green vegetables, specifically the dark green, leafy varieties, activate the T-bet gene, so allowing for the development of a subgroup of cells in the immune system. These cells are known as innate lymphoid cells and play a crucial role in keeping levels of harmful gut bacteria low.

The same research that showed that green vegetables activate the T-bet gene also revealed that saturated fats and refined sugars work to prevent the gene from optimum function.[13] This knowledge gives us a great deal of control over our immune system health!

Greens enhance our spirit and mood

Studies have concluded that a diet high in processed foods and high-fat dairy products is a risk factor for the onset of depression.[14] This can present itself in several forms, but is commonly characterized by a lack of motivation, bouts of sadness, frustration, a disrupted sleep pattern, fatigue, unexplained crying, and irrational thoughts. Something I think we all want to avoid!

When people experience clinical depression, or even just a few symptoms of depression, they can be easily tempted to consume sugary and high carbohydrate foods—or comfort foods, as they are better known. Any satisfaction from doing so is short lived and can exacerbate the problem. This is because these foods cause irregular blood sugar levels, leading to a bad mood and a craving for more junk foods.

Those following a diet with a high intake of green vegetables are less likely to suffer depressive symptoms than those who don't. Research suggests that sufferers of depression often have high levels of homocysteine in their blood.[15] Folic acid, however, can help keep levels of homocysteine low and green vegetables are a fantastic source of it. All women of childbearing age and pregnant women in the first trimester are also advised to take folic acid to prevent any neural defects developing,[16] but they too can also benefit from its depression-reducing properties.

Greens improve liver and kidney function

Your liver is responsible for over 400 various functions in the body. The liver aids in the digestion of food, the storage of nutrients, and the detoxification of your entire system. Your kidneys also have an important role and are continuously working to clean your blood. In order to persist at optimum function, both of these organs require nourishment from nutrients.

When the kidneys aren't able to filter waste products from the body, toxins begin to build up, which can lead to confusion, weakness, lethargy, and a shortness of breath. As the problem worsens, the kidneys become incapable of removing potassium from the body and that, in extreme cases, can be fatal. Although a nutrient deficiency is unlikely to cause kidney disease, revising your diet to become more nutrient dense, especially in regards to protein intake, can be beneficial toward sustaining remaining kidney function in those suffering from renal failure. It is also, of course, an advisable preventative measure.

As the largest solid organ in your body, the liver is also one of the most important. It is tasked with the mammoth job of converting nutrients from the foods you eat into forms that can be utilized by the rest of your system. The liver is also responsible for producing bile without which your body would be unable to move waste products on to the intestines. Although it is a large organ, the liver can be sensitive and will become stressed easily when it is exposed to a large amount of pollutants or processed, unhealthy foods. For this reason, it is essential to consume foods that stimulate and preserve optimum liver function.

Artichokes are a favorite of the liver due to their high amounts of cynarin, which encourages the existence of bile. Artichokes also contain high numbers of flavonoids, especially silymarin—which causes protective reactions to occur inside the liver itself.

Green vegetables also contain a certain type of antioxidants, known as anthocyanin antioxidants, which can reduce free-radical damage to the liver, also known as oxidative stress. This means that if you are eating a diet high in saturated fat or refined sugars, then it is all the more important to have a high consumption of green vegetables to help to crowd out the bad stuff you are consuming!

Greens clear congestion

Inflammation of the sinuses can be due to a range of things, such as bacteria, pollutants, or a virus, and can lead to intense headaches and blocked nasal passages.

Increasing your intake of quercetin is a good way to combat sinus problems. Quercetin is an antioxidant that is found in abundance in green vegetables and it has some serious anti-inflammatory properties. Consuming large amounts of green vegetables will also improve your immune system overall, which will help to prevent sinus problems and congestion occurring in the first place.

Chronic sinusitis is a problem that more than 37 million Americans suffer with every single year. Far from just causing discomfort, symptoms can include pain in the face and teeth, fatigue, a sore throat, and mucus. Some cases are so severe that they require surgery. However, prevention through diet is achievable.

The tissue lining of the sinuses is protected and maintained by vitamin A, and it is thought that vitamin C can reduce swelling in the sinus region. As we know, green vegetables are a great source of both of these vitamins. Additionally, zinc is a mineral that prevents the growth of infectious viruses in the body. As bad bacteria can often cause congestion, it is a great idea to equip ourselves with all the protection we can in terms of infection-fighting foods. Those with a high zinc count are therefore a sensible choice. Cabbage, Brussels sprouts, and green peas are just three green vegetables that have a particularly high zinc count.

A peek at spinach and why you'll want to eat it

I am sure most of us were brought up with parents who told us that we needed to eat our spinach because it is good for us and because Popeye ate it, too! But did any of us know why? I know I didn't. I just thought I might get big muscles like Popeye! So here is my spinach 101 for you.

Spinach is an excellent source of phytonutrients, which are known to keep the body healthy and protect against diseases. It is very low in calories with 1½ cups (100g) of raw leaves providing approximately just 23 calories, and therefore especially useful in controlling cholesterol and aiding weight loss.

The majority of vegetables contain a selection of phytonutrients but spinach is practically at the top of the class when it comes to phytonutrient content. There are at least a dozen different flavonoid compounds in spinach and each boasts important anti-cancer and anti inflammatory properties.[17] Spinach is high in vitamins K, E, C, and A, as well as being a particularly great source of iron and a selection of essential B vitamins.

The high vitamin K content of spinach spells great news for the health of your bones. It can help prevent the breakdown of cells in the bones, while also activating the protein in bones, keeping them healthy. That's not to mention the other nutrients contained within spinach that promote bone health, such as magnesium and calcium. Spinach is second only to kale when considering green vegetables that provide the best dose of vitamin K.

Not only is spinach great for your insides, but also amazing for your skin, and upping your intake is a good natural remedy if you suffer with dry, flaky skin.

When shopping for spinach, choose leaves that look vibrant and fresh. If the leaf looks like it is starting to lose its vitality then it will contain fewer nutrients than the fresher looking leaves. As the leaves age, even slightly, the vitamin C count drops, as does its levels of phytonutrients, so avoid buying it in this state. Generally spinach is super easy to find, super affordable, and super worth it!

A peek at kale and why you'll want to eat it

Kale is a similar species of plant to cabbage and is classed as a green, cruciferous vegetable. It contains high levels of vitamins K, C, and A, as well as a host of minerals such as phosphorous, manganese, iron, and potassium. Gram for gram, kale has more than twice the amount of vitamin C than an orange! And they say that kale is the queen of Vitamin A as it provides 133 percent of the RDA of vitamin A. It is incredibly low in calories while also being high in protein—yes protein! It is one food that without a doubt has earned the superfood label.

Kale is one of the world's healthiest foods and is absolutely crammed full of goodness. Like other dark leafy greens, it is amazing for your bone health, as well as your hair and skin. Kale is a particularly good plant-based source of iron if you are following a meat-free diet. Plus, its use in improving blood glucose levels, preventing cancer,[18] and lowering blood pressure have all been explored extensively with encouraging results.

Just one cup (70g) of kale contains only 33 calories but has nearly 3g of protein and nearly 5g of fiber. Kale also contains omega-3 fatty acids. Although the omega-3 count of kale is low in comparison to other animal-based sources, such as fish, it is a great way to reach your quota if you are following a plant-based diet. Omega-3 fats are essential for optimum health as they promote cardiovascular function, manage cholesterol levels, and are also thought to have an impact on the behavioral development of children.[19] But for me, it is all about the calcium.

> A single serving of kale has more absorbable calcium than a small carton of milk.

Can you believe that the average American only eats two to three large handfuls of kale every year? Don't you think that's rather sad, considering the amazing and awesome health benefits of kale? Luckily, there are a many varieties to choose from and it is also not difficult to grow kale in your vegetable plot, if you have one— meaning you can enjoy the amazing health benefits of this food at a low price. So there should be NO excuses for not getting kale into your diet, right?!

A peek at Swiss chard and why you'll want to eat it

Swiss chard is an absolute powerhouse of nutrition containing high levels of vitamins K, C, and A, as well as a wealth of iron, potassium, and magnesium. A single large handful of this delicious green vegetable will provide a massive 300 percent of your recommended daily intake of vitamin K. That same handful will only pack approximately 35 calories, making it a win-win situation.

Swiss chard contains at least 13 various antioxidants, including flavonoids that are especially useful at protecting the cardiovascular system. One of the most important flavonoids in Swiss chard is called syringic acid and is known to be a great weapon for regulating blood sugar. It is able to do this by inhibiting the activity of an enzyme that restricts the amount of carbohydrates that can be broken down into simple sugars. When this restriction is lessened by syringic acid, it is easier for the enzymes to do their job properly and so leads to steadier blood sugar levels. Ongoing research is taking place to determine the use of syringic acid in treating and preventing diabetes.

Swiss chard also contains unique types of phytonutrients known as betalains. These particular phytonutrients are great for providing anti-inflammatory, antioxidant, and detoxification support to the entire body.

Many nutrition experts consider Swiss chard to be close behind spinach and kale in its nutritional value. The vivid color of Swiss chard, both of the leaves and the stalks, signifies a very rich and dense presence of valuable phytonutrients, while its high levels of calcium, magnesium, and vitamin K make it an excellent source of bone support, too.

When cooking Swiss chard it is always advisable to boil it first in order to free up the acids inside and create a sweeter taste. However, it's important to discard the cooking water, rather than use it in your food preparation, due to its high acid content.

A peek at broccoli and why you'll want to eat it

Broccoli is particularly high in soluble fiber and that means good things for your digestive system, as well as for lowering levels of LDL cholesterol. The fiber in broccoli binds with bile acids in your digestive system, making it easier for the bile to be excreted from the body. This in turn leads to lower LDL cholesterol levels.

It also has a high count of omega 3 fatty acids, which are great for tackling inflammation, among other things, in the body. The collective anti-inflammatory effects of broccoli are known to be good for repairing damage within the blood vessels, which contributes toward improved circulatory health.

This cruciferous vegetable is an especially concentrated source of vitamin C, which means positive things for a great number of functions in the body. It gives you a boost to help fight off colds, as well as reducing the toxicity of medications and chemicals. Broccoli aids the synthesis of collagen, which is not only great for your skin but also important for the structure of blood vessels, tendons, ligaments, and bones. Broccoli also contains high levels of flavonoids that help the body to reuse existing vitamin C stores.

As broccoli is high in fiber and considered to be a good carbohydrate, it will leave you feeling fuller while also preventing constipation and helping to maintain low blood sugar. Broccoli is also known to aid your body in the natural detoxification process due to its special combination of three glucosinolate phytonutrients, which assist all steps of the detoxification process.

Vitamin D is one of the only vitamins that I recommend should, in some cases, be taken as a dietary supplement. However, broccoli could be your secret weapon in tackling vitamin D deficiency. That is because prominent levels of vitamins A and K work to keep vitamin D stores balanced, and there are especially high numbers of both these vitamins in broccoli.

Your digestive system is going to reap the benefits when you increase the amount of broccoli in your diet. There is approximately 1g of dietary fiber in every 10 calories of broccoli meaning that you don't have to eat much to enjoy the healthy rewards. Not only is the function of the digestive system improved by dietary fiber, but it also better equips that part of the body to support the good bacteria that exist there.

As we get older our eyes, too, are affected by the aging process and it's something that a great many people experience at some point in their lives. However, our diet can help protect our sight. Two carotenoids that are present in broccoli, known as zeaxanthin and lutein, have an important role to play in maintaining optimum vision. The retina in particular relies on a strong concentration of lutein to keep it functioning properly.

Just be mindful not to overcook broccoli because when this happens, you will not only lose the flavor and texture but also a great deal of the nutritional value.

A peek at cabbage and why you'll want to eat it

This round, leafy green vegetable is used in cooking throughout the world and with so many health benefits it's easy to see why. It is great for preventing headaches, treating stomach ulcers, clearing up skin disorders, and makes a useful part of a weight-loss program.

Just like broccoli, if your diet is lacking in vitamin C then cabbage can help to rectify the situation. Comparatively, cabbage contains more vitamin C than oranges, and can be cooked and eaten in many different ways. A lack of vitamin C can be responsible for signs of premature aging due to its role in helping to prevent and treat damage to the cells of your body.

Cabbage is also rich in fiber and therefore a fantastic source of roughage. If you don't get enough of this in your diet then you may suffer with constipation and the secondary problems associated with it, such as bloating and, worse case scenario, bowel obstruction. With an adequate amount of fiber in your diet your body will be able to retain more water and help the food to move through your intestines and bowel smoothly.

But my favorite attribute of cabbage is the good bacteria it deposits in our good bacteria bank! Good bacteria are fantastic for our digestion, immune system, fighting candida, reducing inflammation, and eradicating yeast infections. A new study at Leiden University in the Netherlands suggests that good bacteria might also be a way to fight anxiety or depression, meaning that good bacteria in the gut may even affect your mood positively![20]

So, without having to take a probiotic in pill form, how can we naturally get these good guys in? It is, in fact, very simple and cabbage is the answer. Believe it or not, most countries around the world have their own special cultured vegetable, from sauerkraut to pickles to kimchi. Include some cultured cabbage, a.k.a. sauerkraut, in your diet every day and you will most certainly reap the amazing benefits!

Seven recipes that include green leafy vegetables

Here are seven fabulous and, of course, simple recipes to get you going on your journey to getting that ONE green leafy veg into your diet every day. You'll also notice that I reference using pink Himalayan salt quite a bit, but don't stress at all if you don't have it! Good quality sea salt works equally well, it's just the pink stuff has extra bonuses. Pink Himalayan salt comes from the stretch of mountains that give it its name and it is thought to have been protected from modern-day pollution by a layer of lava. It contains more than 80 minerals, as well as being rich in iodine, which is why I prefer to use it in my cooking.

Carrot and Cannellini Bean Curry

A gorgeous twist on your typical curry, this creamy and spicy recipe hits the spot on those cold winter days.

Makes 2–3 servings

- 1 tbsp coconut oil
- 1 medium onion, finely diced
- 1 large sweet potato, peeled and cubed
- 3 carrots, peeled and cubed
- 14fl oz/400ml can of coconut milk
- 1 tsp ground turmeric
- 1 tsp ground cumin
- 1 red chili, deseeded and finely chopped

2 cups/16fl oz/450ml vegetable stock

14oz/400g can of chopped tomatoes

14oz/400g can of cannellini beans

2 cups/5oz/140g fresh spinach, roughly chopped

Place the coconut oil in a large skillet (frying pan) on a medium-high heat. Add the onion and gently sauté for 5–6 minutes, stirring often, until softened and starting to caramelize.

Add the sweet potato and carrots, and continue to sauté for a further 8–10 minutes, stirring often. Next, add the coconut milk, turmeric, cumin, and chili, and cook for a further 2–3 minutes, stirring occasionally.

In a separate pan, on a high heat, bring the vegetable stock to the boil. Add the vegetable stock to the skillet and stir well to combine. Bring to the boil for a couple of minutes then reduce the heat to a gentle simmer.

Add the tomatoes and cannellini beans and leave to simmer for a further 15 minutes.

Finally, add the spinach in the last 2–3 minutes of the cooking time.

Serve immediately either on its own or with your choice of grain.

Kale and Winter Vegetable Soup

This hearty soup is filled with all of my favorite veggies and provides a fantastic blast of tasty nutrients.

Makes 6–8 servings

2 pints/1.2L vegetable stock

1 butternut squash, peeled and cubed

1 sweet potato, peeled and cubed

1 cup/6oz/175g broccoli, chopped

½ cabbage, finely shredded

2 medium carrots, peeled and diced

1 tbsp coconut oil

1 large onion, finely chopped

6 garlic cloves, peeled and minced

4 cups/10oz/280g kale, finely chopped

A handful of fresh cilantro (coriander), trimmed and coarsely chopped plus a few extra sprigs for garnishing

Place the vegetable stock in a large soup or stockpot on a high heat and bring to the boil. Then add the butternut squash and sweet potato and leave to cook for about 10 minutes, or until the root vegetables have softened. Next add the broccoli, cabbage and carrots to the soup before reducing the heat to a gentle simmer and leaving to cook for about 5–6 minutes.

In a separate skillet (frying pan), on a medium-high heat, heat the coconut oil. Add the onion and garlic to the skillet and gently sauté for about 5–6 minutes, stirring often, or until the onions are soft and starting to caramelize. Cooking the onion and garlic separately this way allows them to release all their beautiful flavors.

Add the onion and garlic to the soup along with the kale and the cilantro (coriander). Leave to cook for about 3–5 minutes. Remove the pan from the heat and blitz the soup to a creamy but fine consistency, either using a handheld blender, food processor, or blender. Return the pan to a low heat and continue to cook for another couple of minutes while stirring to ensure that the soup is smooth and combined.

Leave the heat down low for a few more minutes and stir gently to make sure all the ingredients have blended properly.

Ladle the soup into bowls and garnish with a sprinkling cilantro (coriander) before serving.

Mushroom Stuffed Cabbage Rolls

Perfect for a snack or an appetizer for a dinner party, these rolls are stuffed with all good things and are so easy to make!

Makes 8–10 rolls

For the rolls

1 small white cabbage

For the filling

1 tbsp coconut oil

1 medium white onion, finely chopped

1 garlic clove, peeled and minced

2 cups/5½oz/150g button mushrooms, washed finely chopped

Pinch of pink Himalayan sea salt

For the sauce

1 tbsp coconut oil

1 clove garlic, peeled and minced

3 large tomatoes

1cup/2½oz/70g spinach

2 cups/16fl oz/450ml cold water

Remove 8–10 outer leaves from the cabbage—being careful not to damage the leaves as you do so. Bring a large pan of water to the boil on a high heat before adding the cabbage leaves. Leave to cook for a few moments then reduce the heat. Leave the pan on a low heat for a further 2–3 minutes or until the leaves have softened. Drain the cabbage leaves and set aside on paper towel to cool and dry.

To make the filling, heat the coconut oil in a skillet (frying pan) set on a medium-high heat. Add the onions and garlic to the pan and cook for 2–3 minutes, stirring gently. Next add the mushrooms and sprinkle over the sea salt. Cook for a further 3–5 minutes. Remove from the heat and blitz with a handheld blender, or in a food processor, for a few moments or until smooth.

To make the sauce, heat the coconut oil in a large skillet, or wide-bottomed saucepan, set on a medium heat. Add the garlic and gently sauté for 3–5 minutes. Place the tomatoes and spinach in a food processor and blitz for a few moments or until smooth. Add the tomato and spinach mixture plus the water to the pan, stir through to combine and leave to simmer on a medium-high heat for 8–10 minutes, making sure to stir frequently.

Assemble the rolls by placing a tablespoon of the mushroom mixture onto each cabbage leaf, making sure to leave about 1in (2.5cm) around the edge. Then roll each of leaves around the filling to create rolls.

Once all the rolls are ready, use a pair of tongs or slotted spoon to carefully place the rolls into the pan of sauce, taking care to ensure that the seam of each roll is facing downwards to keep the rolls closed.

Leave to cook in the sauce on a medium heat, occasionally drizzling with sauce. After 10 minutes, reduce the heat and allow the rolls to simmer for a further 10 minutes.

Place the rolls on a plate, drizzle over with the remaining sauce, and serve immediately. To make this dish more of a main meal, serve the cabbage rolls on a bed of brown rice.

Quinoa Stuffed Green Peppers

If you're feeling the need for greens then I highly recommend this tasty recipe, as it's loaded with green leafy veg and full of flavor.

Serves 4

- 4 green, red, or yellow bell peppers
- 1 tbsp coconut oil
- 1 small onion, finely chopped
- 3 garlic cloves, peeled and minced
- 1 stalk celery, finely chopped
- 1 cup/8oz/275g Swiss chard, shredded
- 2 medium tomatoes, finely chopped
- 2 cups/13oz/375g quinoa, cooked to packet instructions
- 1 cup/5½oz/150g cashew nuts

A handful of fresh spinach, chopped

1 tbsp fresh parsley, trimmed and chopped

Preheat the oven to 425°F/220°C/gas mark 7.

Cut the tops off the peppers and set aside, then scoop out and discard the seeds so that the peppers are ready for filling.

To make the filling, heat the coconut oil in a skillet (frying pan) set on a medium-high heat before adding the onion, garlic, celery and Swiss chard, and sautéing for about 5 minutes. Add the tomatoes and cooked quinoa and continue to cook for a further 2 minutes. Finally add the cashew nuts, spinach, and parsley, and cook for a further 2 minutes, stirring gently to combine.

Spoon about 2 tablespoons of the mixture into each of the peppers, and then continue to fill all of the peppers until each is stuffed to the top, then replace the stem so that the peppers retain their moisture while cooking.

Place the stuffed peppers on a non-stick baking tray, cover with aluminum foil, and bake in a preheated oven for 20–25 minutes.

Serve with a green salad plate and enjoy.

Green Vegetables in Curried Coconut Sauce

This tasty green curry is aromatic, creamy, green, and a tad bit spicy—absolutely delicious and heartwarming.

Serves 2

1 tbsp coconut oil

1 onion, chopped

2 garlic cloves, peeled and minced

½in (2.5cm) fresh ginger, peeled

1 cup/6oz/175g broccoli, chopped

1 cup/5½oz/150g green beans, sliced

½ cabbage, finely shredded

1 leek, sliced

1 tsp ground cilantro (coriander)

Pinch of cayenne pepper

½ tsp ground turmeric

½ tsp ground paprika

2 cups/5oz/140g kale, shredded

14fl oz/400ml can of coconut milk

Pinch of pink Himalayan sea salt

Heat the coconut oil in a large skillet (frying pan) on a medium-high heat for a couple of minutes before adding the onion, garlic and ginger and gently sautéing for 2–3 minutes, or until the onion is soft and starting to caramelize.

Add the broccoli, green beans, cabbage, and leek and stir gently to combine. Next sprinkle over the cilantro (coriander), cayenne pepper, turmeric, and paprika together with a splash of water if necessary. Cook for 5–10 minutes before adding the kale and cooking for a further couple of minutes.

When the kale begins to wilt, reduce the heat and add the coconut milk. Leave to simmer for about 5 minutes before finally seasoning with sea salt to taste. Serve on its own or with the grain of your choice.

Simple Sauerkraut

Homemade sauerkraut is much better than store-bought versions, which often contain preservatives, and is jam-packed with good bacteria.

Makes 10 servings (16oz/1lb Mason Jar)

- 1 medium cabbage
- 1 tbsp caraway seeds
- 1 tbsp pink Himalayan sea salt
- ½ cup/2oz/60g carrot, grated

Remove about 4–6 of the larger outer leaves from the cabbage and set aside. Next, core and shred the rest of the cabbage.

Place the shredded cabbage with the caraway seeds, sea salt, and carrots in a large bowl and, using your hands, massage the mixture for about 10 minutes to combine the ingredients and allow all the juices to be released.

Once the juices have been released, spoon the mixture into a 16oz/1lb Mason jar and then press or pound the mixture down into the jar until the juices come up and cover the cabbage. Leave about 2in (5cm) of space at the top.

Place the whole cabbage leaves over the mixture—this ensures that the sauerkraut remains airtight. Seal the jar firmly with the lid.

Keep the Mason jar at room temperature covered with a tea towel for three days and then transfer to your refrigerator. The sauerkraut is now ready to eat but you'll find that it improves over time! It will keep for up to two months in the refrigerator.

Spicy Kale Chips

Munch out on this super-healthy snack that has all the crunch of potato chips (crisps) and is packed with all the good stuff but none of the bad.

Serves 2-3

1 big bunch of kale

1½ tbsp almond butter

1 tbsp olive oil

½ tsp ground cumin

½ tsp chili flakes

½ tsp pink Himalayan sea salt

Preheat the oven to 350°F/180°C/gas mark 4.

Wash and dry the kale, dry completely, then tear into large pieces, being sure to remove the thick stalks. Set aside.

In a large bowl, mix together the almond butter, olive oil, cumin, chili and sea salt until well combined.

Place the kale leaves into the bowl and toss in the almond butter mixture until all the leaves are evenly coated.

Spread the kale leaves on a non-stick baking tray and bake in a preheated oven for 10–15 minutes or until crisp.

Eat straight from the oven or store in an airtight container for up to three days.

Chapter 2

Get Heart Healthy
with Whole Grains

Learn how and why to include quinoa, millet, brown rice, oats, and buckwheat easily and effortlessly in your diet every day.

Whole grains are made up of the bran, the germ, and the endosperm. These are all three parts of the grain kernel, making it an entire grain. The outer covering, known as the bran, is the shell, which is tasked with protecting the seed. The bran is a rich source of minerals, fiber, and many B vitamins. The germ is where the embryo of the plant lives and is therefore a serious source of many vitamins, minerals, and other nutrients. The germ is also a rich source of unsaturated oils. Finally, the endosperm is the largest part of the kernel and provides the energy for the seed to grow.

Before humans learned to grind grain, they would eat it straight from the stalk. This meant that our ancestors were consuming a food that was high in fiber and full of vitamins, minerals, antioxidants, and phytochemicals.

It wasn't until late in the 19th century that industrialized roller mills came into use and a process called milling was used to refine the grain. The process of milling removes the bran and the germ from the grain, thereby making it easier to chew. The removal of the germ means that all the goodness contained within is lost. However, it also means that the storage time is prolonged due to the removal of the unsaturated oils, which can go rancid without proper refrigeration.

Although refining grains produces fluffy flour that is perfect for making light pastries and breads, the nutritional sacrifice is huge! Nearly all of the vitamin E is removed during milling, along with at least half of the B vitamins and practically all of the fiber.

Whole grains contain fiber

Whole grain foods are a great source of dietary fiber, while most refined grains contain very little fiber at all. Dietary fiber is important primarily because it helps to reduce LDL cholesterol levels while also improving heart health. Heart disease is a serious problem that kills more than half a million Americans every year. In fact, heart disease is so prevalent that it is the number one cause of death in the USA. That's scary news and is among many other reasons to take care of your heart health with your diet.

An advantage of obtaining fiber through whole grains is that when you do so, you are likely to feel much fuller than if this source of fiber is absent from your meal.

There are two different types of fiber, soluble and insoluble, and they're both valuable in keeping your digestive health in tip-top condition.

Soluble fiber helps to keep glucose levels and blood cholesterol low, while insoluble fiber keeps food moving through the digestive system, preventing constipation. The noticeable difference between the two is that soluble fiber dissolves in water whereas insoluble fiber does not. Whole grains are an amazing source of fiber but it can also be found in beneficial amounts in legumes, nuts, fresh fruits, and vegetables.

Research has shown that increasing your daily intake of soluble fiber, by 5–10g per day, you could decrease your LDL cholesterol levels by 5 percent.[1] Between 20–30g of fiber per day is the preferable and recommended amount. Research has also shown that people who eat a diet rich in whole grains tend to have higher levels of good cholesterol (HDL cholesterol) and lower levels of LDL cholesterol in general. We discuss this in more detail later.[2]

It is interesting to observe that fiber is in fact a type of carbohydrate that the body is incapable of digesting. For this reason it passes through the body undigested but, in doing so, it helps to regulate the use of sugar in the body while also keeping blood sugar levels and hunger under control.

To get more fiber into your diet, aim to include a wide range of whole-grain foods by substituting white rice and bread with whole-grain varieties.

As well as protecting against heart disease, fiber also helps to prevent the onset of diabetes. People who eat a diet containing numerous foods that cause sudden increases in blood sugar are at a high risk of developing type 2 diabetes. As dietary fiber helps to prevent erratic blood sugar levels, it can be an effective weapon in combating this disease.

Whole grains aid digestion

Your digestive tract is one part of the body that can particularly benefit from the nutritional value of whole grains. Because whole grains contain all three layers of the grain (the bran, germ and endosperm) they contain a wide range of beneficial nutrients. These nutrients, alongside the fiber previously discussed, are amazing for intestinal health.

Eating a high-fiber diet helps to relieve pressure in the intestines, which can in turn protect against diverticular disease. When diverticular disease occurs, pouches are formed in the colon which then leads to irritation and swelling. Complications can also occur, which can lead to rectal bleeding.

It has been suggested by experts that to enjoy optimum digestive function you should eat at least 50 percent of your grains as the whole grain variety.

If you are not currently eating a diet that is rich in whole grains, then it is important to introduce these foods slowly to avoid bloating and gas. Your system will soon get used to your new dietary regime and these problems will not persist if done properly.

If you are allergic to gluten or suffer from gluten intolerance then there are several whole grains that you can eat without suffering the ill effects of many other grains. For example, brown rice, quinoa, amaranth, buckwheat, millet, and flax are all gluten free.

Whole grains help to lower cholesterol

Your cholesterol numbers are determined by the amount of cholesterol that is carried by three fat-transporting chemicals in your body, known as lipoproteins. One of these, called low-density lipoprotein, or LDL, moves cholesterol through your body and delivers it to your cells. That is why we refer to LDL as the bad cholesterol. The good cholesterol count comes from the high-density lipoprotein, or HDL, as this is what takes cholesterol away from the cells. The third lipoprotein is known as very-low-density lipoprotein, or VLDL, which carries both cholesterol and fats around the body. VLDL can often turn into LDL when a certain amount of fat is released.

High levels of LDL cholesterol in the body increase the risk of several diseases and health problems. Although a number of factors, such as age, gender and overall health affect your cholesterol level, your diet also plays an important role.

The LDL cholesterol will often merge with fat, calcium, and other substances in the blood to form a waxy, plaque-like substance. The danger from LDL cholesterol comes as this plaque builds up in the walls of the arteries as it impairs the flow of blood to the heart and brain. This build up also makes the arteries less flexible and can lead to a blood clot. There are no physical symptoms of having too much bad cholesterol in your body, making it all the more risky to let your numbers get too high. Blood clots are extremely dangerous and can often be fatal.

Studies have shown that increasing your intake of whole grains may help to lower your LDL cholesterol levels and decrease your risk of ill health.[3,4]

It is thought that the high antioxidant content of whole grains is the reason for it being so good at keeping cholesterol levels under control. Although antioxidants can't directly lower your cholesterol levels, they can restrict the amount of harm that LDL cholesterol is able to cause. While LDL cholesterol is building up as plaque in the walls of the arteries, it can become exposed to free radicals, which then leads to bigger problems. A high presence of antioxidants in the system will prevent the LDL cholesterol from being negatively influenced by free radicals.

Whole grains contain an abundance of antioxidants known as polyphenols. These antioxidants are proven to have a wide range of health benefits, not least their impact on LDL cholesterol damage.

Whole grains lower blood pressure

A diet that is high in whole grains can, in some instances, be as effective as medication when it comes to controlling blood pressure. Low blood pressure can cause you to feel nauseous and high blood pressure leads to disease. Medium blood pressure should be the aim and when you achieve it you will feel energized and healthy. When you control your blood pressure your risk of developing serious health problems, such as renal failure, aneurysm, and heart problems, becomes much less.

Studies have shown that consuming three servings of whole grains every day can greatly reduce blood pressure.[5,6] Keeping your blood pressure low will help to prevent the onset of hypertension, an elevation of the blood pressure in the arteries. Hypertension massively increases the risk of heart disease and stroke. Although three servings would be the optimum amount, studies have also shown that you can still enjoy the benefits of whole grains in smaller amounts.[7,8] Therefore if you are able to even include one whole grain food in your diet each day then you will still be making an incredibly positive change. These benefits are brought about by the impressive nutrient count contained within whole grain products. As the bran and germ still remain, whole grain foods are able to nourish the body in ways that refined grains simply can't.

Potassium has especially strong links to lower blood pressure and is found in high levels in whole grain foods. The only real reason for avoiding foods that are high in potassium is if you suffer with kidney problems. However, if this doesn't apply to you then you can enjoy many benefits from a high-potassium diet, especially when followed at the same time as a low-sodium diet.

Not only can eating whole grains prevent high blood pressure in the first instance, but they can also help to reverse existing blood pressure problems. One in three adults (29 percent of the population) suffers with high blood pressure in the USA. That amounts to 70 million Americans.[9]

Whole grains aid weight loss

A diet rich in whole grains has been shown to help shift excess weight. It seems that belly fat is a particular target of whole grain foods and studies into the effect of whole grains on abdominal fat have had encouraging results.[10,11]

Not only can incorporating whole grains into your diet lead to weight loss, but also eating refined grains can cause weight gain. People aim to lose fat for different reasons but an increased risk of ill health and certain diseases should be the priority of these reasons. Extra body fat, especially in excessive levels, can cause all kinds of health problems, which can then be hard to get under control.

The great thing about whole grains is that they are incredibly filling without being bad for you. Choosing to try whole grain foods also encourages new meal ideas—and that is great for staying motivated in terms of choosing healthy options.

If a meal hasn't satisfied your appetite then you're more prone to snack, which can lead to weight gain. However, if you do need to eat between meals and you're "watching your weight" then try popcorn because it's a fantastic, low-fat, whole-grain snack. Not only is popcorn full of nutrients, but it is also quite filling, which means you tend to eat less overall. Of course, the weight loss potential of snacking on popcorn is hindered if you add toppings to it. However, a light sprinkle of salt or a natural sweetener can increase the flavor without compromising on calories.

Whole grains are quite low in calories when compared to refined grains. That means that you can eat until you are full without being too concerned that you have overdone it.

Whole grains help maintain steady blood sugar levels

The amount, and types, of carbohydrates you eat largely impact your blood sugar level—also referred to as your blood glucose level. As we know, whole grains contain high amounts of fiber, which cannot be broken down by the body. For that reason, this fiber doesn't bring any calories into the body and neither does it raise blood sugar levels.

Studies have shown that people who suffer with diabetes are much better able to control their blood sugar levels when they consume adequate amounts of whole grains.[12-14] Experts have long been suggesting that replacing refined simple sugars with more complex food sources is the best way to prevent diabetes occurring in the first place. Research has shown that this decrease in risk is greater than 16 percent in most instances, even when just one whole grain is included in the diet.[15]

When refined starches, such as white rice, white bread, or in fact anything that contains white flour, enters the body it will act similarly to sugar when the body starts to digest it. This means that blood sugar levels will spike causing havoc in the blood system. Therefore, avoiding refined starches is as important as avoiding refined sugar.

Although there are two types of fiber—soluble and insoluble—it is the soluble variety that has an influence over blood sugar levels.

However, a large amount of soluble fiber has to be consumed in order to benefit from this. When whole grains are embraced, it won't be hard to reach this level of soluble fiber in the diet and you will soon start to reap the benefits.

If you are not eating at least 20g of fiber a day, then you should definitely consider upping your intake. Men tend to need more fiber than women so if you are male and experiencing erratic blood sugar levels, then this is all the more important.

Whole grains make you feel fuller longer

As we have touched upon briefly already in this chapter, it is mostly the fiber in whole grains that leaves you feeling full. The obvious intention of wanting to feel fuller for longer is for weight loss. A diet that incorporates low-calorie, high-fiber foods is perfect for weight loss as it means an adequate amount of food can be consumed without fearing weight gain.

Insoluble fiber is the type of fiber that works best at keeping you full for longer. That is because instead of dissolving in water like soluble fiber does, it absorbs the water, which then creates a feeling of fullness in your stomach. This water absorption also adds moisture to stools, making constipation much less likely. Whole grains in general are a great source of insoluble fiber.

Eating a combination of protein, complex carbohydrates, and unsaturated fats will also help to leave you feeling full for longer.

This is because your blood sugar is considerably stabilized by these components, which also add to your energy stores. Protein is an especially important factor as it promotes satiety while also helping your body to burn more calories and fat than it would with depleted stores. Proteins are also thought to keep you fuller for longer, which of course will mean you will want to eat less.

When you consume protein and fiber in the same meal, your body digests them slower than it would if you ate them alone. The longer the process of digestion takes, the longer you will go without feeling hungry again.

Eating a high-fiber, high-protein food with each meal will ensure that you feel satisfied after a sensible-sized portion. The whole grains mentioned in the following part of this chapter are all fantastic choices and will leave you feeling full while also nourishing your body with the goodness it needs.

A peek at quinoa and why you'll want to eat it

Quinoa is a high protein, gluten-free whole grain that is available in a range of colors—the most popular varieties are red, black, and white. The difference between the colors is more in the texture as opposed to the taste or the nutritional value. White quinoa is fairly fluffy when cooked whereas the black and red varieties are crunchier and less likely to clump together.

Quinoa is an Andean plant that is most commonly found growing wild in Bolivia and Peru. The Incas prized the grain as far back as 4,000 years ago and it featured heavily in their diet. The Spanish tried to restrict the cultivation of this amazing grain during the European conquest, scorning it as a food of the Indians, but luckily for us they were unsuccessful and its popularity continues to increase.

The high protein count of quinoa is additionally impressive because it contains nine of the essential amino acids that are required for optimum nutrition. It is rare for this number of essential amino acids to be found in the same plant-based food source. There is only approximately 200 calories in one cup (185g) of cooked quinoa, and it is favorably high in iron and fiber, as well as being a great source of magnesium.

Before you cook quinoa it is advisable to rinse it in order to rid the layer of the protective substance that coats the grain. It is not uncommon to find pre-rinsed quinoa in the grocery store, but if you are unsure then there is no harm in rinsing it before you begin cooking.

Quinoa is cholesterol free and exceptionally low in fat with just 3.4g of fat in each cooked cup (185g). Its use in preventing cardiovascular illnesses, among a range of other diseases, is huge and no doubt will be the subject of further research and studies.

A peek at millet and why you'll want to eat it

Millet is a very small grain, which can either be gray, white, red or yellow. Hulled millet is the most popular kind although the cracked variety is also available in stores.

Millet is particularly popular in Africa and Asia and practically all millet production takes place in these continents. It grows quickly, even in dry, hot conditions, making it the perfect grain for these regions.

Millet contains more than 80 different nutrients making it an incredibly healthy choice. Of those nutrients, copper, phosphorous, magnesium, and manganese are among the most important. It is one of the best choices of grain when it comes to considering your heart health. This is due in large part to the high amounts of magnesium contained within. Magnesium has been proven to lower high blood pressure and also lowers the potential for heart attacks.

The high level of phosphorus in millet is also a great reason to include it in your diet. Phosphorus is absolutely essential in maintaining the body and so a deficiency means optimum health is impossible. This mineral contributes to every single cell in the body and is particularly important for forming strong teeth and bones.

A peek at brown rice and why you'll want to eat it

During the production of brown rice, only the very outer layer, the hull, is removed, which means very little damage is done to the nutritional value of the grain. However, when brown rice is milled into white rice, over 70 percent of the nutrients are lost. This loss of goodness means that many varieties of white rice are now required to be fortified with certain vitamins. That, of course, is no substitute for the real thing and whole grain brown rice is always going to be your best option!

It is thought that rice was first cultivated over 6,000 years ago in China. However, this idea has recently been disputed as archeologists believe they have found farm tools, which appear to have been used for planting rice, dating back over 9,000 years.

Brown rice is a fantastic source of manganese, niacin, magnesium, copper, phosphorus, and selenium. Manganese is important as it helps the body to produce energy from the carbohydrates and proteins that we eat. It is also an essential ingredient for maintaining a nervous system that operates at optimum function. Niacin, also known as vitamin B3, works to lower cholesterol and promote cardiovascular health. Magnesium has several important jobs to play in the body such as lowering blood pressure, preventing migraines, and also reducing the risk of many diseases. Without ample supply of copper, the body wouldn't be able to grow properly and the health of all tissue in the body would suffer. With a copper deficiency comes the appearance of premature aging and low energy. The main function of phosphorus in the body is to keep teeth and bones healthy. However phosphorus also impacts how the body uses fats and carbohydrates. Selenium is a trace mineral that has been the subject of much research into lowering the risk of colon cancer.[16] Selenium is also a major contributor to immune system functionality. Also, the oils contained within brown rice lower LDL cholesterol.

The cardiovascular benefits of eating brown rice can be enormous, especially in postmenopausal women. If you fall into this category and already suffer from high blood pressure or high cholesterol, then brown rice can be an effective weapon in the fight back to good health.

A peek at buckwheat and why you'll want to eat it

Buckwheat is actually a fruit seed and is not in any way in the same family as wheat. It is known to be a gluten-free super food! It is an amazing source of protein as well as containing high levels of rutin, which is known to treat high blood pressure. Buckwheat ranks low on the glycemic index, making it perfect for lowering blood sugar levels.

There is slight confusion over the origins of buckwheat. Historically experts believed it to have been from central Asia, near Manchuria, however, recently fresh research has come to light, which suggests that it originated in China and the Himalayan region.[17]

Buckwheat is high in vitamins and minerals but low in calories. Buckwheat also contains healthy carbohydrates, which are used by the body as an effective energy source. As well as being low in calories, it is low in fat and high in protein. This whole grain is a particularly good source of folic acid and other B vitamins.

> The natural properties of buckwheat are perfect for strengthening the intestines, which in turn can improve the appetite.

An advantage of eating buckwheat over other whole grain products is that because it grows so quickly, there is less prevalence of growers using chemicals on it. This of course makes it better for the body than grains, which have been grown with pesticides and chemicals.

A peek at oats and why you'll want to eat them

Oats may not look like the most exciting of food choices but once you understand the nutritional makeup of a bowl of oats, you will soon be keen to include them in your diet.

It is largely thought that oats came about as a mutation of the wild oat plant and the oldest recorded use of oats was in Switzerland during the Bronze Age. They were brought to North America in the early 1600s and continued to grow in popularity in the centuries that followed.

Just one cup of oats (85g) packs an impressive 6g of protein and 4g of fiber. Additionally, just one cup will provide almost 70 percent of your daily recommended amount of manganese—an essential mineral for bone formation. The same cup of oats is also crammed full of magnesium and vitamin B1, but less than 150 calories.

Oats have the highest soluble fiber count of all of the whole grains, making it the best choice for keeping your LDL cholesterol low. Oats also pack a healthy dose of insoluble fiber making them good for boosting your digestive health, too.

Oats are usually just thought of as a breakfast option, but they are also great for using baking, cooking, and adding to smoothies. They can bring texture and additional nutrition to foods that might be lacking it.

Far from being a food that is good for your insides, oats also have the right properties to hold moisture and gently exfoliate the skin when applied externally. Mix one cup (85g) of oats with a dash of honey to make a low-cost but effective skincare moisturizing exfoliator.

However, unlike most grains that can be stored for quite some time, try not to buy more than two months' worth of oats at a time, as you are likely to find that they will spoil. Make sure you store them in an airtight container to get the longest shelf life possible.

Seven recipes that contain whole grains

Here are seven of my favourite recipes to get you going on your journey to getting whole grains into your diet every day.

Quinoa and Red Pepper Chili

The quinoa gives this dish all the lovely "meaty" taste you'd expect from chili without the meat!

Serves 2–3

2 red bell peppers

2 red challis

1 tbsp coconut oil

1 cup/7oz/200g zucchini (courgettes), diced

1 large onion, finely diced

2 large tomatoes, finely chopped

4 garlic cloves, peeled and minced

1 tsp ground cumin

½ tsp paprika

Pinch of ground chili powder

1¼ cups/10fl oz/280ml vegetable stock

½ cup/3oz/100g quinoa, uncooked weight

400g/14oz can of pinto beans, drained and cooked

½ cup/4fl oz/125ml water

Pinch of pink Himalayan sea salt

Wash the red peppers and challis then cut them in half, lengthwise, making sure to remove and discard all of the seeds.

Place the peppers and challis on a baking tray and place under the broiler (grill) on a medium-high heat for 10 minutes. When they are softened and slightly charred, but not burned, remove them from the broiler and cut into small chunks.

Heat the coconut oil in a large saucepan on a medium-high heat for a couple of minutes before adding the zucchini (courgettes), onion, tomatoes and garlic. Sauté the vegetables in the coconut oil for a few minutes before adding the cumin, paprika, and chili, and sauté for a further minute. Finally add the red peppers and challis you prepared earlier, and stir gently to combine.

Add the vegetable stock, quinoa, pinto beans, and water to the saucepan then bring to the boil. After a few moments, reduce the heat and simmer for a further 20 minutes, or until the quinoa has absorbed all the vegetable stock.

Serve immediately and enjoy.

Quinoa with Carrots and Button Mushrooms

Quinoa is one of the fastest-cooking grains and I think one of the tastiest! Here's a quick and easy but, of course, nutritious meal, which is the perfect recipe for those days when you don't have a lot of time.

Serves 2-3

1 pint/568ml vegetable stock
Pinch of pink Himalayan sea salt
1½ cups/9oz/250g quinoa, uncooked
1 tbsp coconut oil
1 large leek, finely sliced
2 carrots, peeled and finely sliced
2 cups/8oz/225g button mushrooms, washed and halved
A handful of fresh parsley, trimmed and chopped
Pinch of freshly ground black pepper

Place the vegetable stock in a large pan with the sea salt and bring to the boil on a high heat before adding the quinoa. After a few minutes, reduce the heat and simmer with the lid on for 10–15 minutes.

In a large skillet (frying pan) heat the coconut oil on a medium-high heat for a couple of minutes. Adding the leeks and carrots and gently sauté for 5 minutes. Add the mushrooms to the skillet and reduce the heat and continue sauté for a further 5 minutes.

When the quinoa has absorbed all the liquid, add the parsley and season with black pepper and stir gently to combine.

Divide the quinoa equally between the serving bowls and top with the mushrooms and vegetables. Serve immediately.

Breakfast Millet

When you want to add a greater variety of grains into your diet, millet is a great choice and it makes the perfect porridge for breakfast. It contains a wealth of essential nutrients, including magnesium, manganese, and copper.

Serves 1-2

2 cups/16fl oz/450ml water

1 cup/7oz/200g of millet, uncooked weight

1 cup/8fl oz/225ml nut milk

¼ cup/1oz/25g pumpkin seeds

Drizzle of maple syrup

Handful of your favorite berries

Place the water in a large saucepan on a high heat and bring to the boil before adding the millet. Reduce the heat to low and leave to simmer for 15 minutes, remembering to stir occasionally.

Add the nut milk and continue to cook on a low heat for 5 minutes, while stirring. Remove the pan from the heat and stir in the pumpkin seeds.

Divide the millet between servings bowls and drizzle with maple syrup. For an extra added antioxidant boost, top with your favorite berries (personally, I love blueberries with this one) and serve immediately.

Kale and Brown Rice Soup

The added grain in this soup makes it more of a one-pot stop. If you don't have brown rice then add quinoa or millet instead — which are also fast-cooking grains.

Serves 2–3

- 1 tbsp coconut oil
- 1 onion, diced
- 3 carrots, peeled and cubed
- 1 sweet potato, peeled and cubed
- A handful of fresh cilantro (coriander), trimmed and chopped plus a couple of sprigs for garnishing
- 1 pint/568ml vegetable stock
- 14oz/400g can of chopped tomatoes
- 1 cup/7oz/200g brown rice, uncooked
- 2 cups/5oz/140g kale, roughly torn or chopped
- Pinch of pink Himalayan salt
- Pinch of freshly ground black pepper

Place the coconut oil in a large saucepan on a high heat to warm for a couple of minutes before adding the onion, carrots and sweet potato. Sauté gently, making sure to stir frequently, for about 5 minutes or until the vegetables have softened and browned a little.

Add the cilantro and the vegetable stock and stir well to combine before adding the tomatoes, kale, and brown rice. Turn the heat down to medium, season with salt and black pepper, stirring continuously.

Place the lid on the pan and leave to simmer for about
20 minutes until the rice is cooked.

Divide the soup between serving bowls, garnish with cilantro
(coriander) and serve immediately.

Honey Nut Oatmeal

The roasted nuts make all the difference to this simple oatmeal
dish, which is packed full of tasty flavor and slow-release
carbohydrates for an energy-filled day.

Serves 2

- ½ cup/2oz/55g mixed nuts
- 4 tbsp organic runny honey
- 1 large banana, peeled and sliced
- 1 cup/8fl oz/225ml nut milk
- 1½/5½oz/150g cups oatmeal

Preheat the oven to 350°F/180°C/gas mark 4.

In a large bowl, combine the nuts and honey. Spread the mixture
over a baking tray covered with greaseproof paper and bake in a
preheated oven for 15 minutes.

When the mixture has browned and the honey is sizzling, remove
from the oven and set aside to cool.

Place the milk and oatmeal in a medium pan and cook on a
medium heat for 5–6 minutes. Add the slices of banana and leave
to cook for a further minute. Remove the oatmeal from the heat

and gently stir in the honey and nut mixture. Drizzle with a little more honey before serving.

Buckwheat Flatbread with Hummus

My kids love this one! Making your own flatbread and hummus is super easy and makes for a great snack or light lunch.

Serves 4

For the flatbread

1 tbsp fresh yeast

1 cup/8fl oz/225ml water

1 tbsp maple syrup

1 cup/4½oz/150g whole grain flour

¾ cup/3oz/115g buckwheat flour

1 tsp pink Himalayan salt

1 tbsp coconut oil

For the hummus

2 cups/12oz/350g chickpeas, cooked and drained

4 cloves garlic

2 tbsp lemon juice

2 tbsp tahini

½ tbsp coconut oil, melted

Pinch of pink Himalayan salt

Pinch of freshly ground black pepper

1 tbsp sesame seeds (optional)

1 tbsp extra virgin olive oil (optional)

To make the flatbread, combine the yeast, water and maple syrup in a large bowl. Add the whole grain and buckwheat flour, and sea salt and combine to create a stiff dough, adding a little more flour if it's sticky before kneading with the heels of your palms for about 3–5 minutes.

As soon as you have a firm, dry dough, place it on a floured board, then cut into four equal parts and roll each part into a ball. Using a pastry brush, lightly cover with coconut oil and then leave in the refrigerator for 2 hours.

Remove from the refrigerator and sprinkle a handful of flour over the balls and then flatten before placing them under the broiler (grill) on a medium-high heat for approximately 5 minutes, or until golden.

While the flatbread is baking, place the chickpeas, garlic, lemon juice, and tahini in a blender and whizz for about 2 minutes, or until smooth. Then add the coconut oil a couple of drops at a time, while blending, to ensure all the ingredients are well combined. Finally season with sea salt and black pepper to taste.

Spread the hummus onto the flatbreads and return to the broiler 5 more minutes.

Top with a sprinkling of sesame seeds and a drizzle of olive oil and serve immediately with perhaps some black and green olives.

Broccoli and Cauliflower Pilaf

Cruciferous vegetables such as broccoli and cauliflower have unique nutritional properties compared to other vegetables because they're packed with phytonutrients—potent anti-cancer agents.

Serves 2-3

    1 tbsp coconut oil

    4 cloves garlic, peeled and minced

    ½ cup/3oz/100g cauliflower

    ½/3oz/100g cup broccoli

    1in (2.5cm) fresh ginger, peeled and minced

    2 cups/14oz/400g brown rice, cooked to packet instructions

    1 tsp ground turmeric

    1 tsp of turmeric

    1 tsp of ground curry powder

    1 tsp ground chili

    1 tbsp ground cilantro (coriander)

    ½ cup/2¾oz/75g cashew nuts, chopped, to garnish

Place the coconut oil in a large saucepan on a high heat to warm for a couple of minutes before adding the garlic and then gently sautéing for 2–3 minutes.

Add the cauliflower and broccoli and continue to cook for 10 minutes, or until it becomes slightly crisp.

Finally add the ginger and brown rice to the pan then stir in the turmeric, curry powder, chili, and cilantro (coriander).

Reduce the heat and cook on a low heat for a further 10 minutes, adding a splash of water if the mixture becomes dry.

Divide between plates, garnish with cashew nuts, and serve immediately.

Chapter 3

Out with Refined Sugars, In with Natural Sweeteners

Learn how and why to include honey, brown rice syrup, maple syrup, date sugar, and coconut palm sugar or nectar easily and effortlessly in your diet every day.

Sugar, sugar, sugar—who doesn't love it, right? It is everywhere and in everything and, a long time ago, we thought that was a good thing, or at least not that bad of a thing. But the more we consumed processed and packaged foods, the more refined sugar we started to consume as well, and in turn the more sick we became. In the past few years we have seen a particularly massive increase in type 2 diabetes, which is just the beginning for a whole host of serious health problems.

For me the greatest gift of quitting sugar is that it helps you to run away from processed and packaged foods too. Why? Because it's been proven over and over again, that sugar is addictive. And once we become addicted, well, frankly, we crave sugar and want it in everything—in particular, everything that comes in a packet! And why is that? Simple, the food industry is super-clever and they know sugar is addictive. Once we are addicted, we tend to buy into the big branded food companies who flavor all of their packaged foods with all that nasty stuff. And that is how they make their money. Nice one, guys!

However, it is possible to avoid playing into their hands. You can choose a diet that is not only free from the processed, packaged foods, which are marketed to us 24/7, but also to live a life free from refined sugars. This is certainly a case of "easier said than done," but once you make the move toward this healthier lifestyle, and you watch your health soar, you will never look at a chocolate bar the same way again. Before you attempt to make such a change, read on to discover just what sugar has been doing to you and will indeed continue to do, should you continue to consume it. At the same time, you'll discover all the benefits of embracing natural alternatives; learn why your body needs the good, and why it definitely does not want the bad!

Refined sugar can make us age faster

Excessive refined sugar consumption has long been linked to premature aging. When excessive sugar consumption is combined with a nutrient-deficient diet, which also includes high amounts of refined carbohydrates, this problem becomes all the more prevalent. The term "glycation" refers to the process linking sugar consumption with early signs of aging: a chemical process that occurs when blood sugar levels experience extreme spikes.

When blood sugar levels are excessively high, the sugar molecules move around the system and bind themselves to other components, creating new formations known as protein-sugar complexes. Funnily enough, these protein-sugar complexes are also known as advanced glycation end products or (funnily enough) AGE for short! Anyway, when these complexes are created, they have a free rein to roam around the body where they induce an inflammatory response, which then leads to tissue damage, which is then responsible for premature aging.

There are molecules in your face that are responsible for keeping your skin from becoming loose. They are incredibly sensitive to sugar and will fail to do their job properly if you follow a diet that is high in refined sugars. Essentially, the sugar attacks the collagen in your skin, which then has a detrimental effect on its elasticity. This, of course, will cause signs of aging to occur. As well as affecting the elasticity of your skin, sugar can also cause the skin to dry and can also acne to develop. The acne problem is due to the effect of sugar on insulin production, which then causes a hormonal imbalance. Every time we consume sugar, the pancreas sends insulin out into the body to counteract it. When the pancreas is doing this too often, because we are eating too much sugar, insulin resistance begins, which is also a serious risk factor for diabetes.

It is possible to reverse the damage to your skin that sugar has caused by eating foods that are high in anti-glycation antioxidants, such as apples, tomatoes, lentils, and beans.

In the past 40 years, sugar consumption in the USA has increased by more than 40 percent, with the average American eating an incredible 2½ pounds (1.15kg) of sugar every week.[1-3] Excess sugar is added to a huge number of processed foods and soft drinks, making it near impossible to monitor your sugar intake if you are consuming products from either of these groups.

Refined sugar can cause obesity

Obesity has more than doubled in the last 30 years and this has happened side by side with a dramatic change in eating habits. Meal portions are growing and fast food has become more popular. With this move toward convenience, we have sacrificed our health and sugar is now being consumed at a rate never before recorded in human history.

For many years, experts believed that fat was the main culprit in the obesity epidemic. However, more and more evidence is continuing to come to light that supports the idea that refined sugar is to blame.

Sugar is often compared to controlled drugs in research,[4] in the sense that it is extremely addictive and incredibly damaging to the body. It is also comparative in the sense that we need to be weaned off it, in order to work toward restoring optimum health.

As discussed above, too much insulin production can be a trigger for obesity. The storage of excess energy as fat cells is due to the hormone insulin and so an increase in its production will inevitably cause chaos in the body.

The problem in eradicating sugar from the diet to combat obesity comes when people continue to eat processed foods. Years ago many people started to avoid high-fat foods on the advice of diet experts and so low-fat options were created. But in order to preserve the flavor of these foods, more sugar was added. What's more, added sugar is not always labeled as such and can be hidden behind a range of different chemicals or carbohydrates, all of which are essentially refined sugar. Fructose is one of the biggest problems when it comes to varying types of sugar found in processed foods. Added fructose in food should certainly be avoided at all costs when trying to lose weight.

It is an undisputed fact that in countries where the consumption of sugar is higher, obesity rates and the incidence of diabetes is also higher. Although optimum health is easier to achieve with the complete eradication of sugar, consuming a small amount will not present too much of a problem. The liver is perfectly capable of metabolizing a reasonable amount of refined sugar each day but that amount has to be limited to just a couple of teaspoons. Therefore sugar, as a treat as opposed to a daily component of the diet is the attitude to adopt, if you want to protect your body and speed up weight loss.

Some immediate steps to take might include avoiding sweetened beverages, reducing your alcohol consumption, and choosing to eat whole fruits instead of drinking fruit juices. Sweetened beverages massively up our sugar intake without providing any nutritional benefit to the body. Alcohol has the same effect on insulin levels as sugar, so is also best kept to a minimum. Finally, fruit juice made from concentrates has practically none of the fiber found in the fruits themselves. Therefore either making fresh juice yourself at home, or checking the labels on the back to make sure it's 100 percent real juice, or simply sticking to eating whole fruits are all healthier choices.

Refined sugar can cause insulin resistance

Type 2 diabetes is becoming increasingly prevalent, and it is estimated that more than 300 million people in the world now have the disease. As described earlier, a poor diet high in sugars and a sedentary lifestyle can lead to insulin resistance and a heightened risk of type 2 diabetes.

Fructose and glucose are the two most prominent components of sugar. The difference between the two is that glucose can be made by the body and metabolized by all cells in the body. However, fructose can only be metabolized by the liver and isn't produced naturally.

When a large amount of fructose is present in the body, then it is turned to fat. Some of this fat is transported in the blood and the rest remains in the liver. Over time this can lead to liver disease and the liver to become insulin resistant. An insulin-resistant liver means elevated levels of insulin in the rest of your system, which over time can lead to obesity and the onset of disease As time goes on, the pancreas will no longer be able to make enough insulin to properly provide glucose to the cells. At this point, diabetes will have already developed.

It has to be noted that fructose from fruit does not cause the same problems as fructose from refined sugar. When consumed from fruit, fructose poses no threat to the body. The exception to this rule is if you are already diabetic, in this instance you should talk your medical practitioner or dietician about how much fruit to include in your diet.

Sugar and labels: How to read them

Understanding the labels on the foods you eat is essential, if you are to truly understand what you are putting into your body.

One teaspoon of sugar is the equivalent of 4g, and presently the average American consumes 20–22 teaspoons of added sugar every day. Checking the labels on foods before buying them is a great way to avoid eating too much. When you consider that 22 teaspoons of sugar is a massive 350 calories, then it's easy to see how weight can be dramatically affected by added sugar.

If a product lists sugar as the first or second ingredient on the label then you are definitely better off not eating that food. Ingredients are generally listed by weight, so if sugar is first then put it back and step away from the shelf! But you also need to know that sugar can be disguised under other names on the label. Alternative artificial sweeteners are becoming more popular with food manufacturers and unfortunately, current laws don't require the manufacturers to specify exactly how much sugar is contained under each names.

Soft drinks are arguably the worst offenders when it comes to added sugar, and worse they offer absolutely no nutritional value. On average, a can of soft drink will contain 150 calories, and the majority of these calories are from sugar. That means there is approximately 10 teaspoons of sugar in each can. Studies have shown that consuming just one can of soda, such as cola, every day can lead to gaining approximately 15lbs (6.8kg) of weight every year[5,6]—and many people drink more than just one!

Breakfast cereal manufacturers also have a lot to answer for when it comes to adding sugar to their products. It is particularly common for breakfast cereal manufacturers to list sugar multiple times under different names. In doing so, the total sugar count becomes near impossible for the average consumer to determine.

Although food labels will often show you, without too much confusion, how much sugar is contained per serving, there is normally little to suggest how much of this is from added sugars, as opposed to naturally occurring sugars.

Here are a couple of common ingredients that you will see frequently on food labels—both the good and the bad!

Glucose

Glucose is the body's favored energy source and it is also known as blood sugar. Most of the carbohydrates that we eat are converted into glucose, which is then either stored in the muscles or liver, or used immediately as energy. Glucose is processed in the gut during digestion and every cell in our body needs the energy that this process creates. Therefore, at adequate levels, glucose is beneficial to cells, but in excessive amounts it can behave like a slow-acting poison and erode cells—especially those in the pancreas that make insulin.

In turn, the pancreas overcompensates for this cell damage by producing too much insulin, which can eventually lead to damage to the pancreas and insulin resistance in the body. High levels of glucose can also cause the blood vessels to harden and narrow, which then compromises blood flow. The consequences of this affects many important and essential functions in the body and can lead to huge problems long term, including kidney disease, nerve damage, erectile dysfunction, vision loss, heart attacks, strokes, poor circulation, and more.

Fructose

This natural sugar is found in small quantities in fruit. However, it is also manufactured in a purer form and added to food and drink products. We need to be particularly wary of fructose because it is metabolized by the liver, bypassing the gut completely, and so produces more fat than other simple sugars. Although some fructose will be stored as glycogen in the body, the majority of it will be turned into fat stores. When fructose is present in the body, it will not prompt insulin to be secreted as it would when glucose is present. In its purest form, fructose is almost 70 percent sweeter than other sugars, making it much more addictive for its taste. Decreasing the amount of fructose in your diet, or eradicating it completely (not including natural fruit), can have a positive impact on weight loss.

Studies have shown that consuming large amounts of fructose can lead to a slower metabolism, high levels of LDL cholesterol, liver disease, heart disease, obesity, and hypertension.[7,8] Fructose also has the dangerous potential to cause leptin resistance in which the body is less able to understand when it is hungry or not, causing us to overeat.

Sucrose

More commonly known as table sugar, sucrose comes from sugar beets and sugar canes, and is also present naturally in fruits and vegetables. Sucrose is 50 percent glucose and 50 percent fructose. When sucrose enters the system, it is converted into separate units of fructose and glucose. The body then treats it as such and it is put to use in the body in the usual way: the glucose is used for energy and the fructose stored as fat. Too much sugar causes the blood sugar levels to spike, which can quickly lead to fatigue and irritability, not to mention tooth decay and a potentially dangerous fluctuation in insulin levels.

High-fructose corn syrup

Sweeter and cheaper to make than other sugars, high-fructose corn syrup is used in abundance in processed foods in the USA— even though it is widely accepted as being bad for our health! In moderate amounts over time, it is known to lead to heart disease, cancer, liver failure, tooth decay, dementia, and obesity. Several studies have been conducted to determine the safety of consuming high-fructose corn syrup, with the results all pointing to the fact that it is toxic for health.[9,10]

Invert sugar

A liquid sugar that is made from fructose and glucose, invert sugar is used widely in commercial food preparation because it helps foods to retain moisture and so extends their shelf life. High in calories without containing any notable minerals or vitamins, it's best avoided.

Malt syrup

Made from malted barley, malt syrup is an unrefined sweetener, and is often used in combination with other sweeteners because, while it isn't incredibly sweet, it does add a malty flavor to foods. Although you will see this ingredient frequently on labels, it is one of the healthier options and nothing to be overly worried about.

Evaporated cane juice

Despite the fancy name, there's not much difference between this sweetener and standard cane sugar. Evaporated cane juice does have slightly more vitamins A, C, and calcium than cane sugar, but that is the only real nutritional difference. It is still 99 percent sucrose and that means empty calories that are not helping your wellbeing.

Refined sugar and addiction

People have long debated whether it is possible to become addicted to sugar and now we are more confident than ever that the answer is a huge YES!

Although this addiction does not have physical traits, as with substance abuse, we are still negatively affected by consuming too much sugar. When the body receives sugar, changes to dopamine levels in the brain are similar to those that happen when people take recreational drugs. Dopamine is the feel-good hormone in the brain and it is released when we undertake gratifying activities, such as eating, sex, and exercise. If levels of dopamine in the brain are low then we will start to crave the activities that will provide it. However, on the flip side, when our levels are too high than addictive behaviors can start to develop. This may ultimately lead to us craving more and more sweet foods without ever really feeling satisfied.

Studies are continuing into the addictive qualities of sugar with recent research published in the *American Journal of Clinical Nutrition* greatly supporting this idea. This research shows foods that cause an excessive elevation of blood sugar to be the most addictive.[11]

If you're guilty of eating certain foods, even when you are not hungry, or the idea of cutting back on these same foods worries you, then the chances are that you are addicted to sugar. If this is the case then you are likely to feel exhausted during the day for no real reason.

Detoxing from sugar might sound like a long process but it is easily achievable within a few days or a few weeks. It is also, of course, possible to go cold turkey from sugar. However, removing sugar from your life slowly is likely to make the transition easier and more successful.

A peek at honey and why you'll want to eat it

Honey is a combination of sucrose and water with enzymes added by the bees themselves. When the bees add their enzymes to the sucrose it converts into glucose and fructose. These enzymes also evaporate much of the water that prevents the honey from spoiling. As the sucrose is naturally occurring, as opposed to commercially processed, it does not have the same damaging effects as table sugar. In fact, in studies conducted to determine the benefit of honey to diabetics, the results demonstrated that honey helped those who took part to lose weight while boosting their good cholesterol levels.[12] If you have diabetes, it goes without saying that you should talk to your medical practitioner or dietician before introducing honey into your diet.

When you break it down, honey is approximately 80 percent glucose and fructose, 18 percent water and the remaining 2 percent is protein, pollen, vitamins, and minerals. The lower the percentage of water in the final product, the higher the quality the honey will be.

There is a selection of amino acids in honey as well as a range of vitamins, including riboflavin, niacin, thiamin, and B6. Honey also contains an extensive range of minerals, including zinc, sodium, potassium, phosphorus, magnesium, manganese, iron, copper, and calcium. A good source of antioxidants, honey is also free from cholesterol and fat. Flavonoids are the particular antioxidant found in honey and they are believed to protect against cancer, as well as reducing the risk of heart disease.[13,14]

Honey has been documented for its medicinal properties as far back in history as the Greeks and the Romans. The Greeks were convinced that honey could increase the lifespan of those who ate it regularly. Today, its use in treating wounds and burns has been explored extensively with positive results. There is also strong research to suggest that consuming a tablespoon of honey each day can help to combat allergies.[15]

Athletes are among those who can also benefit from consuming honey as studies have shown that it can enhance performance and improve recovery time.[16]

A peek at brown rice syrup and why you'll want to eat it

Brown rice syrup, also known as rice malt syrup, is mostly made of glucose, making it a healthy choice as a natural sweetener. A derivative of brown rice, it is made by exposing cooked brown rice to enzymes that turn the starches into much smaller sugars. The thick syrup that is created as a result is incredibly easy for your system to digest and contains trace amounts of certain minerals such as potassium and calcium, while also providing your body with fiber.

> Brown rice syrup doesn't contain any fructose, so it doesn't have the same detrimental effect on the liver, or metabolic health, as other artificial sweeteners.

Brown rice syrup scores fairly low on the glycemic index at around 25. When we consider that refined table sugar ranks at 64, this is clearly the best option for a low-GI diet. The GI or Glycemic Index is a system that rates the carbohydrate quota of the foods we eat. It then shows how quickly each food impacts the blood sugar (glucose) level. So the higher the GI rating, the faster the increase in our blood glucose. As brown rice syrup contains soluble complex carbohydrates, it can take up to three hours to absorb into the bloodstream. During this time your blood sugar levels remain more consistent due its slow-release action, and this can help us maintain our energy levels and be less prone to feeling irritable and tired during the day.

A peek at maple syrup and why you'll want to eat it

This healthy natural sweetener is made from the sap of maple trees and has been consumed for several hundreds of years. The majority of maple syrup, at least 80 percent of it, is made in Canada by drilling a hole into the maple tree and collecting the sap. The sap is then boiled until the majority of the water evaporates, leaving the thick, sugary syrup, which is then filtered to remove any impurities.

When buying maple syrup it is important to purchase the real product rather than maple-flavored syrup. Maple-flavored syrup is much cheaper to produce than actual maple syrup but contains high levels of refined sugars. It will also often contain high fructose corn syrup, which as discussed earlier, can be incredibly detrimental to health.

A general rule is the darker the color of the syrup, the stronger the flavor. The darker syrups are better for baking, the lighter ones better for toppings.

Maple syrup is loaded with minerals and antioxidants, such as manganese, zinc, iron, potassium, and calcium. There are at least 24 different antioxidants in maple syrup, making it great for combating the oxidative damage caused by free radicals. This makes it a great addition to the diet for reducing your risk of disease. The zinc in maple syrup keeps you healthy because when you become deficient in zinc your immune function can become compromised. Maple syrup is also a rich source of vitamins, several of which are essential to the proper function of your cells. The most prominent vitamins in maple syrup are niacin, folic acid, B2, B5, B6, and vitamin A.

A peek at date sugar and why you'll want to eat it

When it comes to the antioxidant count of sweeteners, date sugar is the clear winner. It is one of the healthiest sugars available and that is thanks in no small part to the manufacturing process. It is made from dried dates, which have been pulverized into a fine powder. It is incredibly sweet but it does not melt like regular sugar does, meaning that it can't be used in all the same ways. Because it is so sweet, it is recommended that when you are substituting white sugar for it in a recipe, you only use two thirds of the amount required.

The minimal processing that occurs to create date sugar means that the final product retains much of the nutrition of whole dates. That means this type of sugar is high in fiber while also boasting a range of vitamins, minerals, and antioxidants.

A peek at coconut palm sugar/nectar and why you'll want to eat it

Coconut palm sugar is derived from the sap of the coconut palm tree. It is made in a similar way to maple syrup, with the sap from the tree being drained and then heated while the water evaporates. It is far more nutritious than refined sugars as it retains the goodness from the coconut palm.

Potassium, calcium, zinc, and iron are the most notable minerals in coconut palm sugar, as well as fiber, all of which slow the rate of glucose absorption by the body.

Medical experts have spoken of how coconut palm sugar is low on the glycemic index, meaning that it is fine for people with diabetes to consume in moderation.[17] This kind of sugar provides a slow-energy release meaning your energy levels will be sustained throughout the day as opposed to highs and lows.

Seven recipes that use natural sweeteners

Here are seven fabulous recipes to get you going on your journey to ditching refined sugars and integrating natural sweeteners effortlessly into your diet.

Red Coconut Cakes

Beets are incredibly sweet and that's why they work so well in cake recipes — like a red velvet cupcake but filled with all things good.

Makes 12 cakes

1¼ cups/6¼oz/190g whole wheat (all-purpose) flour

¼ cup/1¾oz/50g coconut sugar

2 tbsp raw cacao

1 tsp baking powder

2–3 large beets, steamed and pureed until smooth

½ cup/6oz/175g organic runny honey

2 tbsp coconut oil

1 tsp lemon juice

1 tsp vanilla extract

Preheat the oven to 400°F/200°C/gas mark 6 and line a 12-cup muffin tray.

Sift the flour, coconut sugar, raw cacao, and baking powder into a large bowl and mix until well combined, and then set aside.

Place the pureed beet, honey, coconut oil, lemon juice, and vanilla extract in a blender or food processor and blitz for 1–2 minutes until smooth. Pour the mixture over the dry ingredients and mix well to combine.

Spoon the mixture into the muffin tray then place in a preheated oven and bake for approximately 20 minutes. After this time, check the muffins have cooked all the way through by inserting a skewer and checking that it comes out clean. If not, return to the oven for another 5 minutes before turning out on to a wire rack to cool before serving.

These cakes stay fresh for three days in an airtight container. Serve with your favorite cup of herbal or green tea and enjoy.

Honey Granola

Granola is such a tasty and simple breakfast choice but store-bought versions are usually laden with sugar! Making a batch at home is the best way to enjoy granola without any of the negative health effects!

Makes 4 servings

1½ cups/5½oz/150g organic runny honey

2 tbsp coconut oil

2 cups/6oz/175g oats

¾ cup/3oz/100g pumpkin seeds

1 tbsp coconut palm sugar

¾ cup/3oz/100g walnuts, chopped

¾ cup/3oz/100g dried dates, chopped

¾ cup/3oz/100g dried apricots, chopped

Preheat the oven to 350°F/180°C/gas mark 4.

Place the honey and coconut oil in a pan on a low heat and until the honey melts.

In a large bowl, mix the oats and pumpkin seeds together then add the melted honey/coconut oil mixture as well as the coconut palm sugar and stir well to combine.

Spread the mixture on to a large non-stick baking tray and bake in a preheated oven for 20 minutes, making sure to turn the mixture every 5 minutes during cooking. Place the walnuts on a separate baking tray and bake in the same oven for 10 minutes.

When the walnuts and the oat mix are ready, place in a large mixing bowl and add the dates and apricots, and combine well. Store in an airtight container where it will remain good for up to a month.

Honey Marinated Tofu with Green Vegetables

A gorgeously sweet supper and quite possibly one of my absolute favorites, as I feel I'm literally energizing my body with as much goodness as possible in one meal!

Serves 2–3

- 1 block of firm tofu
- 1 tbsp coconut oil
- 2 cups/5oz/140g kale, chopped
- 1 cup/6oz/175g broccoli, chopped
- 1 leek, sliced finely
- 1 cup/1oz/25g Swiss chard, chopped
- 1 tbsp coconut oil

For the marinade

- 2 tbsp organic runny honey
- 2 tbsp soy sauce
- ½ tsp chili powder

1 tsp ground cilantro (coriander)

2 cloves garlic, peeled and minced

1 tsp lemon juice

Start by making the marinade. Place all the marinade ingredients in a small bowl and stir well to combine. Cut the tofu into small chunks then place it and the marinade in an airtight container and leave in the refrigerator for 12 hours or overnight.

Place the coconut oil in a large skillet (frying pan) on a medium to high heat to warm for a couple of minutes then add the tofu from the marinade and fry for 5–10 minutes, making sure to turn the tofu pieces regularly so they cook evenly.

Add the kale, broccoli, leeks, and Swiss chard to the pan and continue to cook for a further 10 minutes, making sure to stir frequently.

Serve immediately and enjoy.

Goji Berry Quinoa Bars

These bars make a wonderful on-the-go snack or quick breakfast—and they're full of goodness!

Makes 6 bars

1 tbsp coconut oil

1 cup/6½oz/185g quinoa, cooked

1 cup/5oz/140g almonds, chopped

1 cup/5½oz/150g dried cherries, chopped

½ cup/2oz/55g goji berries

2 tbsp brown rice syrup

½ cup/4fl oz/125ml water

Preheat the oven to 425°F/220°C/gas mark 7 and grease an 8×8×1in (20×20×2.5cm) square bake pan (cake tin) with a light layer of coconut oil.

On a separate baking tray, spread the quinoa and almonds and place in a preheated oven for 10 minutes. When the mixture is toasted, remove the tray from the oven and reduce the heat to 350°F/180°C/gas mark 4.

Place the cherries, goji berries, brown rice syrup and water into a food processor and blitz for 1–2 minutes, or until smooth. Transfer to a large mixing bowl and add the toasted almonds and quinoa. Stir well to combine.

Spoon the mixture into the bake pan and press down firmly with the back of a spoon. Ensure the mixture covers the bottom of the pan evenly. Then place in a preheated oven and bake for 20 minutes.

Once cooked, cut the mixture into bars before turning out onto a wire rack to cool. These bars will keep fresh in an airtight container for up to five days.

Sweet Potato Salad

This simple salad make a filling lunch and sweet potatoes are a healthier alternative to traditional white potatoes, as they have a lower GI and are absolutely brimming with antioxidants.

Serves 2-3

2 sweet potatoes, peeled and diced

½ cup/3oz/100g of quinoa, uncooked weight

1 tbsp coconut oil

1 red bell pepper, deseeded and chopped

3 scallions (spring onions), finely chopped

1 cup/6oz/175g cherry tomatoes, halved

Pinch of pink Himalayan sea salt

A handful of fresh cilantro (coriander), trimmed and chopped

Place the sweet potatoes in a large saucepan and cover with water, bring to boil on a high heat and cook for 20-25 minutes or until the potatoes are soft enough to push a fork through. Drain and set aside.

While the sweet potatoes are cooking, place the quinoa in a separate saucepan and cook as per the packet instructions.

Place the coconut oil in a large saucepan on a medium heat to warm for a couple of minutes, then add the sweet potatoes and sauté for 5 minutes. Next add the red pepper, scallions (spring onions), and cherry tomatoes and cook for a further 5 minutes.

Remove the pan from the heat and add the quinoa and stir gently to combine.

Finally season with sea salt to taste and a sprinkle of fresh cilantro (coriander) before serving.

Quinoa Breakfast Bites

My quinoa breakfast bites are a delicious alternative to refined cereal breakfast options and simply bursting with nutrients! The combination of quinoa with fruits and natural sweeteners make for a dish that is full of goodness and has a pleasing texture.

Serves 2-3

- 1 tbsp coconut oil
- 1 cup/6oz/175g quinoa, uncooked weight
- 1 banana, peeled and thinly sliced
- 1 cup/3½oz/100g blueberries
- 1 tbsp ground cinnamon
- ½ cup/6oz/175g organic runny honey
- 2 cups/16floz/450ml non-dairy milk
- 1 tbsp nut milk (optional)

Preheat the oven to 400°F/200°C/gas mark 6 and grease an 8×8×1in (20×20×2.5cm) square bake pan (cake tin) with a light layer of coconut oil.

Place the quinoa, banana, blueberries, cinnamon, honey and non-dairy milk in a bowl and stir to combine well.

Pour the mixture into the bake pan, place in a preheated oven and cook for about 45 minutes, or until most of the liquid has been absorbed.

Spoon immediately into bowls, drizzle with a little nut milk and enjoy, or simply store in an airtight container for up to a week.

Apple and Raspberry Crumble

This easy crumble makes a fantastic dessert but without all the refined sugar and butter of traditional crumble recipes while tasting just as good.

Serves 3–4

- 1 cup/5oz/150g of whole wheat (all-purpose) flour
- 1 cup/3oz/85g oats
- ½ cup/3½oz/100g date sugar
- ½ cup/1¾oz/50g walnuts
- 1 tsp ground cinnamon
- 2 tbsp maple syrup
- 4 apples, peeled, cored, and chopped into 1in (2.5cm) chunks
- 1 cup/4½oz/125g fresh raspberries
- 1 tbsp lemon juice

Preheat the oven to 425°F/220°C/gas mark 7.

To make the crumble, place the flour, oats, date sugar, walnuts, and cinnamon into a large bowl and mix together well before adding half the maple syrup and mixing again.

Place the apple chunks, raspberries, the rest of the maple syrup, and the lemon juice into a baking dish, ensuring that the fruit is evenly spread over the bottom of the dish.

Sprinkle the crumble mixture evenly over the fruit, making sure the fruit is completely covered by the crumble, then bake in a preheated oven for 1 hour or until the fruit is bubbling and the top is golden.

This crumble is delicious served hot or cold.

Chapter 4

Goodbye Refined Oils, Hello Healthy Unrefined Oils

Learn how and why to include olive oil, coconut oil, and flaxseed oil easily and effortlessly in your diet every day.

Growing up the in the heartland of America, the good ol' Midwest, I'm pretty sure that nearly everything I consumed was cooked in oil. From the French fries to the chicken nuggets to the corn dogs—you name it—and I LOVED it! But back then, we didn't know nearly as much as we do now about how bad processed oil can be for our health.

The 101 on unrefined oils vs. refined oils

The vast health differences between unrefined oil and refined oil are incredibly important to consider when striving for optimum health.

Unrefined oils don't undergo any chemical or filtering processes. There is minimal heat involved in their production and they are not deodorized or bleached in any way after extraction, which means none of the good nutrients are lost. Oils of this kind tend to have a richer flavor and be more nutritious than their refined counterparts.

Extracting oil from plants can be done in many different ways. Refined oils tend to be produced by chemical and heat extraction processes, whereas a method known as cold pressing is generally used for unrefined oils.

Within the category of unrefined oils, there are further terms that explain how many times the fruit, nut, or other ingredient was pressed in order to extract the oil. When an oil is labeled "extra virgin," it means it was only pressed once, whereas a "raw" or "virgin" labeled oil would have undergone the extraction process twice or more.

What's up with the smoke point?

When the temperature of oil is raised above a certain point, its nutritional value and the flavor can be compromised; this temperature is referred to as the "smoke point." It is important to know the smoke point of oils that you are using in order to choose the right oil for the dish you are preparing.

Oils with a very low smoke point should only ever be used cold. That means olive oil is only really suitable for drizzling over foods.

However, if it has been refined then the smoke point will be slightly higher, meaning you could use it for light sautéing. Flaxseed oil should also not be used for cooking, as it too has a low smoke point and best reserved for drizzling over food after cooking or to make things like salad dressings. Coconut oil has a higher smoke point than olive oil and flaxseed oil and it can be used for sautéing, medium heat frying and is also great in baking!

For example, if you want to fry something for a dish, then it is best to choose an oil with a higher smoke point because the hotter the temperature the oil can withstand, the better. If you are planning on using oil for baking, then it is fine to use an oil with a lower smoke point. This is because the dish will be heated slowly, at a less intense heat than using it for other purposes would involve.

The majority of unrefined oils contain high numbers of health-boosting enzymes and minerals; however, these compounds don't always react well to heat. When heated above their smoke point, these oils can become rancid and taste bitter as a result, which is why they are better suited to low temperature cooking or for drizzling over dishes.

Oils with very high smoke points normally undergo several refinement processes to eliminate the naturally occurring enzymes and minerals that won't withstand heat. This results in a refined oil that has a higher smoke point and also a longer shelf life.

When you are cooking with an oil and you exceed its smoke point temperature, it will start to break down and release free radicals, which, as we know, contribute to the aging and degradation of cells. It will also produce a chemical known as acrolein, which leaves food with an acrid, sharp taste and smell, so avoiding oils that create this is recommended.

Being aware of the different smoke points of oils will help to enhance your cooking and to keep all the best nutrients locked in your food.

Composition of fats in oils

Consuming nutrients that have beneficial, health-boosting qualities is essential for the optimum function of our bodies. Monounsaturated fats and polyunsaturated fats are two types of nutritious fats naturally found in oils, and you should aim to include them in your diet.

Monounsaturated fats are known to have beneficial effects on your health when you consume them in moderation. Fats of this type are so called because they have one unsaturated carbon bond in each molecule. Polyunsaturated fats differ from monounsaturated fats because they have more than one unsaturated carbon bond in each molecule.

Fats of this kind are helpful in reducing LDL cholesterol levels and also contain nutrients that are beneficial to cell health. As we discussed earlier, high LDL cholesterol levels can lead to all sorts of serious health problems, so it is best to consume healthier kinds of fats.

Oils that are rich in polyunsaturated fats are great for providing the essential fats, which the body is unable to make on its own, such as omega-3 and omega-6. In order to help you distinguish between them, it is helpful to know that oils containing monounsaturated fats or polyunsaturated fats will generally be liquid when stored at room temperature. They will only become solid if the temperature drops.

Oils that contain monounsaturated fats include olive oil, canola oil, safflower oil, and sesame oil. Oils that contain polyunsaturated fats include soybean oil, corn oil, flaxseed oil, and sunflower oil. Making sure you know the differences between oils helps you make a more informed choice about what you're consuming.

The extraction processes: Refined and unrefined

Refined and unrefined oils go through different processes before they reach the shelves.

Refined oils are made by subjecting the seeds to chemical and mechanical processes to extract oil from them. During these processes, the naturally occurring nutrients are eradicated so the oil oxidizes easily. However, while this means that the oil is easier to cook with, it also means that it is much easier for the oils to be broken down during cooking, which then lets free radicals loose in the body.

In order to make refined oils, the seeds are first collected, cleaned, and crushed. Then they are heated at temperatures of up to 350°F

(180°C) and then put through a press, which uses further heat and friction to extract oil from the pulp of the seeds. The seed pulp then passes through a bath of hexane solvent to extract more oil. It is worth noting that hexane is made when crude petroleum oil is refined and has a range of negative health effects. After the hexane solvent bath is over, the mixture of seed and oil is then separated in a centrifuge. The final stages then involve further refining of the oil such as degumming, neutralization, bleaching, and deodorization.

Consuming refined oils regularly can cause inflammation in the body, which is therefore a contributing factor in serious illnesses, such as heart disease, cancer, and diabetes.

Degumming involves adding water to the extracted oil whereas neutralization involves removing impurities by treating the oil with sodium hydroxide or sodium carbonate. Bleaching serves the purpose of removing any off-color material from the oil and is achieved by adding bleaching agents into the mix. Deodorization is generally the final step during which pressurized steam is used to remove any remaining compounds that might be detrimental to the final product.

Unrefined oil isn't subjected to any of the above processes and instead only undergoes a light filtration to remove any large particles present. This chemical-free process, called expeller pressing, works by mechanically compressing the seeds and so forcing out the oil.

Why you'll want to throw away these refined oils

The main reason why refined oils are so bad for us, and really not worth keeping in the cupboard, is that they contain acids and fats that negatively affect our health. There is also the issue of genetic modification—as most of these oils have been produced from GM plants—which could also potentially be harmful to health.

For example, canola oil—made from extracting the oil of rapeseed plants—contains trace amounts of erucic acid. This acid has been shown to cause heart damage during studies of its effect on animals.[1] Other studies have also demonstrated that consuming certain amounts of canola oil can cause a vitamin E deficiency in the body.[2,3]

Corn oil is one of the biggest culprits of genetic modification and as a result has lost some of its more natural benefits. Further consider that it has then gone through all that refining and you have a recipe for a health disaster.

> Refined oils add excess fats and acids into your diet so, by avoiding them, you'll ensure that your body only absorbs the best nutrients.

A peek at coconut oil and why you'll want to eat it

Coconut oil contains a unique combination of fatty acids that are known to be extremely beneficial for our health. These fatty acids are called medium chain triglycerides and are metabolized differently than other saturated fats. These fatty acids move quickly from the digestive tract to the liver where they serve as an energy source.

Regularly eating coconut oil can be effective for weight loss, especially when it comes to losing abdominal fat. It also helps to boost the immune system, increases energy, and encourages healthy hair growth. Your skin also has a lot to gain from either regular consumption or regular topical application. This is mostly because coconut oil has absorptive qualities that will retain moisture in the skin but also because of the wealth of vitamins and minerals contained within it. When applied topically, coconut oil also provides natural defense against the sun and can be used in place of sunscreen in moderate heats.

Research has shown that fats of this kind are useful in preventing and combating the symptoms of certain brain disorders. Studies indicate that those suffering with Alzheimer's could see particular benefits, as coconut oil provides an alternative source of energy for cells by increasing the level of ketones in the blood. This then assists the cells that are failing to function properly in the brains of Alzheimer's sufferers.[4,5]

Medium chain triglycerides increase energy expenditure in the body, which means the calories you are eating get used up quicker than with other kinds of fat. This makes it great for those looking for a lower calorie oil to use in cooking.

The fatty acids contained within coconut oil are also known to lower levels of LDL cholesterol in the body while improving HDL cholesterol levels. I know I have mentioned this before but I can't stress it enough—reducing LDL cholesterol levels greatly reduces the risk of heart disease and stroke!

Although coconut is seen as a health food in the West, there are several cultures around the world that consider it to be a staple of their diet. These cultures have thrived for many generations and do not suffer from the same high levels of ill health and obesity seen in the West.

A peek at extra virgin olive oil and why you'll want to eat it

Extra virgin olive oil is a staple fat in many diets, most famously the Mediterranean. A great deal of research has been conducted to determine the health benefits of consuming this oil. These studies have concluded that the fatty acids and antioxidants in olive oil have powerful health benefits and regular consumption is recommended.[6,7]

Olive oil is made from pressing olives and while this is a simple process, it is sometimes done using a chemical extraction process or diluting olive oil with other oils. It is important to make sure that the olive oil you purchase is pure and made in the right way for the best benefits to be experienced.

Extra virgin olive oil is the best option because the label means it has been extracted using natural methods. It will have a very distinctive taste and will contain high numbers of antioxidants as well as beneficial amounts of vitamin E and vitamin K.

Chronic inflammation is a huge contributing factor to many prevalent diseases, such as cancer, heart disease, diabetes, arthritis, and Alzheimer's disease. Extra virgin olive oil is known to fight inflammation in the body due to its high antioxidant count and the presence of oleic acid. For this reason, regular consumption of this kind of oil can help to protect the body over time from these diseases. Studies have also shown that olive oil is useful in protecting against cardiovascular disease and strokes.[8, 9]

As well as fighting inflammation, extra virgin olive oil works to prevent oxidative damage to LDL particles and so can protect us against heart disease. It is also best at preventing blood clots and improving the quality of blood vessel linings. Additionally, studies have shown that patients with high blood pressure can dramatically reduce their need for medication by increasing their consumption of extra virgin olive oil.[10]

A peek at flaxseed oil and why you'll want to eat it

Flaxseed oil, also known as linseed oil, contains a wealth of health-boosting compounds. Flaxseed has been cultivated for over 7,000 years, originally in Europe but now all over the globe. Throughout this time, it has been valued for its medicinal qualities, proving to have uses in treating inflammation and digestive complaints.

The essential fatty acids in flaxseed oil are the main reason why it is such a great source of health. These essential fatty acids help to make improvements across the entire body, protecting cells from damage. These fats also help to prevent against heart disease and other illnesses. Just one teaspoon of this oil every day provides an ample amount of the omega-3 and omega-6 needed to keeping the body running at its best. Several studies have shown that regular consumption of flaxseed oil can also help lower cholesterol and regulate blood pressure.[11,12]

Sufferers of lupus have also found flaxseed oil to be of particular use in relieving symptoms. Not only does it reduce any inflammation in the joints or kidneys but also its cholesterol-lowering properties are useful. This is because high cholesterol is thought to be a trigger for elevating this disease.

The high levels of dietary fiber in flaxseed oil make it great for digestion and preventing or treating constipation. Those who are afflicted by bowel disease can use this oil to help repair any intestinal tract damage. It is also thought that flaxseed oil helps to prevent gallstones from developing in the body.[13,14]

Your insides are not the only part of you that can benefit from flaxseed consumption. Your skin, hair, and nails will experience the benefits as well. The essential fatty acids are useful in treating skin conditions such as eczema and rosacea, and the oil itself can be used externally to treat sunburn. When it comes to your hair and nails, it is again the fatty acids that are responsible for the nourishment. They help to promote healthy nails and revitalize hair.

Seven recipes that include these good oils

Here are seven fabulous and, of course, simple recipes to get you going on your journey to getting healthy, unrefined oils into your diet every day.

Roast Carrot and Cannellini Bean Salad

I love this salad because it's just so different! You have your greens from the Romaine, your lovely vitamin-A rich carrots, protein from your beans, and omega-3 from your oil! Sounds pretty perfect to me.

Serves 4

6 large carrots, scrubbed and peeled

2 tbsp coconut oil, melted

1½ cups/5½oz/150g green beans

1 onion, finely diced

1 Romaine lettuce, roughly torn or shredded

400g/14oz can of cannellini beans, drained and washed

1 cup/6oz/175g cherry tomatoes

1 tbsp olive oil

Pinch of pink Himalayan sea salt (to taste)

Pinch of freshly ground black pepper (to taste)

Preheat the oven to 400°F/200°C/gas mark 6.

Place the carrots in a roasting pan, rub with the melted coconut oil and roast in a preheated oven for 30 minutes.

Blanch the green beans by placing them in a large pan of boiling water for 2–3 minutes, before draining and rinsing with cold water. Set aside.

In a large bowl, place the onion and lettuce, cannellini beans, and cherry tomatoes and combine gently.

When the carrots are cooked, chop them finely before adding them to green beans and seasoning with sea salt and pepper to taste.

Divide into serving bowls, drizzle with olive oil, serve, and enjoy.

Olive Oil Baked Sweet Potatoes

As you can probably tell from some of the other recipes in this book, I love my sweet potatoes because they are packed full of antioxidants and this humble jacket potato recipe makes for the perfect and simple lunch.

Serves 4

4 medium sweet potatoes, scrubbed and peeled

1½ tbsp olive oil

1 tsp ground cumin

1 tsp ground, smoked paprika

Pinch of pink Himalayan sea salt

Pinch of freshly ground black pepper

Preheat the oven to 425°F/220°C/gas mark 7.

Slice each of the sweet potatoes lengthwise into six pieces of equal size.

Place the sweet potatoes on a baking tray, drizzle with olive oil, and sprinkle with the cumin, smoked paprika, sea salt, and pepper then place in a preheated oven and leave to bake for 30 minutes.

Halfway through cooking, remove the potatoes from the oven and turn them to ensure they bake evenly.

Serve alone or with your favorite salad!

Raw Coconut Balls

If you're a coconut junkie, then this will be your go-to snack.
Packed with superfoods and natural sweeteners, this recipe will
also help keep any sweet cravings in check.

Makes 10-12 balls

2 cups/7oz/200g desiccated coconut (plus extra for rolling)

2 tbsp coconut oil

2 tbsp raw honey

1 tsp lucuma powder

1 tsp chia seeds

Place all the ingredients in a blender and blitz for 2–3 minutes or
until you have a thick, coarse mixture.

Remove the mixture from the blender and, using a large melon
baller or your fingers, scoop and shape the mixture into 10–12 balls.

Roll each of the balls in a little desiccated coconut, and place in
the refrigerator to chill for about 20 minutes before serving.

This tasty treat will stay fresh in your refrigerator for up to
three days.

Spicy Stir-fried Broccoli

I love spice and always say the spicier the better, so this recipe is my kind of spice! Rather than boiling or steaming the broccoli, we are going to sauté it in a lot of good-for-you coconut oil.

Serves 4

3½ cups/9oz/250g soba noodles

5 tbsp coconut oil

2 medium onions, diced

700g broccoli, chopped into small florets

2 cups/5½oz/150g mushrooms, cleaned and chopped

1 lime, juiced

1 tsp chili flakes

Pinch of pink Himalayan sea salt (to taste)

Pinch of freshly ground black pepper, to taste

Cook the soba noodles according to the packet instructions.

Place the coconut oil in a large skillet (frying pan) on a medium heat to warm for a couple of minutes then add the onion and sauté gently for 2–3 minutes.

Next add the broccoli and continue sautéing for approximately 5 minutes before adding the mushrooms. Reduce the heat to low and cook for a further 5 minutes, stirring regularly.

Add the juice of the lime to the pan and then sprinkle the chili flakes over the top. Continue to cook for a further 5 minutes.

Serve over the soba noodles and enjoy immediately.

Kale and Spinach Pesto

A wonderful twist on the classic pesto! Filled with three amazing greens and using flaxseed oil instead of the traditional olive oil.

Serves 4

2 cups/5oz/140g kale

2 cups/5oz/140g spinach

2 cloves garlic, peeled

3 tbsp of almonds

2 tbsp flaxseed oil

A handful of fresh cilantro (coriander), trimmed and chopped

1 tbsp lemon juice

½ tsp pink Himalayan sea salt

½ tsp freshly ground black pepper

Place all the ingredients in a blender and blitz for 2–3 minutes, adding more flaxseed oil or lemon juice if necessary to reach your preferred consistency.

Serve with your favorite pasta! I love quinoa and corn pasta but my kids prefer whole wheat, so take your pick and enjoy.

Spicy Coconut Rice

This is a great dish on its own but you could add some tofu to make it more hearty. However you choose to eat it, it's a great way to spice up some rice.

Serves 4

- 2 tbsp coconut oil
- 2 cloves garlic, peeled and minced
- 1 red onion, diced
- 2 cups/5oz/140g kale, roughly chopped
- 2 cups/5oz/140g spinach, roughly chopped
- 2 tbsp chili flakes
- 2 cups/14oz/400g brown rice, cooked to packet instructions
- 1 cup/3½oz/100g desiccated coconut
- Juice of 1 lime

Place the coconut oil in a large skillet (frying pan) on a medium heat to warm for a couple of minutes. Add the garlic and red onion and sauté for 5–6 minutes, stirring frequently, until the onions start to caramelize.

Add the kale and the spinach and leave to cook for 5 minutes, stirring frequently before adding the desiccated coconut in too, stirring, and leaving to cook for a further minute.

Add the cooked rice and stir well. Drizzle the juice of the lime over the top and sprinkle over the chili flakes. Cook for a further 3–5 minutes.

Divide onto plates, garnish with a little cilantro (coriander) and serve immediately.

Flaxseed Pancakes

Getting omega-3 into you diet by eating oils couldn't be easier with this super yummy pancake recipe. Light, fluffy, and utterly delicious!

Serves 2

> ½ cup/5oz/150g whole wheat (all-purpose) flour
>
> 2 tbsp flaxseed oil plus extra for cooking
>
> 1 tsp baking powder (bicarbonate of soda)
>
> ¼ tsp baking soda
>
> ½ cup/4fl oz/125ml dairy-free milk
>
> 2 tbsp maple syrup

Place all the ingredients in a large bowl and beat until the mixture forms a smooth batter.

Drizzle a little flaxseed oil into a small skillet (frying or pancake pan) set on a medium heat.

When the oil is hot, pour about 2–3 tablespoons of the batter into the skillet so that it covers the bottom of the pan in a thin layer. Turn the pancake after approximately 4 minutes and cook the other side. Repeat with the rest of the batter.

Drizzle with a little more maple syrup and top with your favorite berries or slices of banana. Serve immediately.

Chapter 5

Get the Fat on Good Fats

Learn how and why to include avocados, nuts, and seeds easily and effortlessly in your diet every day.

When I tell people that I eat a half an avocado pretty much every single day... they often look pretty shocked and I can hear them thinking, "... but avocados are full of fat!" So you can imagine their faces when I say that I also eat a very small handful of nuts and a sprinkle of seeds on a daily basis too. What gives these foods such a bad rap is the word "FAT". We have been brainwashed into thinking that all fats and everything that contains fat is just super bad for us, and we will then in turn, become that word... fat! But I am here to tell you with my hand on my heart, that some fats are very, very good for you, in fact, great for you!

Here is the simple lowdown: We need fat to function at our very best, but I am talking the whole food kind of fat. Fat from whole foods help make our skin look radiant and supple. Fats lubricate our joints, which then keep our yoga/running/walking/exercising in tip-top form. Fats even protect our cells from oxidative damage. But we also need fats to help absorb a lot of nutrients that are fat-soluble. For example, vitamins A, D, E, and K need good fats in order to be properly absorbed by the body. We have discussed oils and the fats in oils in the previous chapter, so this one is more about the fats in whole foods. I am just going to break it down for you and keep it simple!

Trans fats

Trans fats are a type of unsaturated fat that occurs from two different sources. The first is formed naturally in the stomach of some animals and therefore finds its way into several animal products, such as meat and dairy. The second is formed during food production when hydrogen is added to vegetable oil. This is done to increase the shelf life, flavor, and texture of many foods.

There is absolutely no nutritional or health benefit to consuming these trans fats, however, there is a lot of harm to be done!

Trans fats are bad for us because they raise LDL cholesterol levels in the body. And, as you know, a high level of LDL cholesterol spells bad news for our health, especially heart health. Heart disease is a leading cause of death and not eating trans fats can massively help when it comes to avoiding this disease.

Research has also found links between trans fats and Alzheimer's disease, cancer, and even infertility.[1-4]

The biggest culprits for a high trans fat count are fast food, fried foods, pastries, cookies (biscuits), pies, frozen dough products, and microwaveable snack foods. It really pays to check the labels of the foods that you are buying so that you know how much of this type of fat you are bringing into your kitchen or your body. If you can see that a product contains hydrogenated oils, or partially hydrogenated oils, then you are better off leaving it on the shelf. It is also a good idea to avoid all processed snack foods.

It is also important to know that just because a food label reads 0g of trans fat, that it doesn't necessarily mean that there is no trans fat in the product! In the USA, this is because regulations state that if a product has less than 0.5g of trans fat per serving, then it can be labeled as having zero. In the UK, there is currently no requirement for trans fat levels to be included on food labeling. Again, this is why it is best to steer clear of processed foods and opt for natural, wholesome options instead.

Saturated fat

Saturated fat is frequently referred to by experts as one of the biggest dietary causes of high blood cholesterol. It is also thought to be a huge risk factor in strokes and heart disease. On the scale of how bad certain types of fat are for you, trans fat is certainly worse than saturated fats but neither are things you should aim to include extensively in your diet.

The scientific definition of a saturated fat is a fat molecule that has no double bond between carbon molecules. This is because they are saturated with hydrogen molecules. What does that mean, you might ask? Well, in regards to your health it essentially means you are going to be eating a high-calorie, high-cholesterol food that is of no real benefit to you!

Recently more research has come to light that suggests saturated fats in small amounts are not harmful for health.[5] However, we must also consider that many foods that contain saturated fat also contain trans fat, additives, and added sugars. Therefore keeping consumption of saturated fat to a minimal amount is still advisable.

The contradiction to this opinion on saturated fat is when it comes to the saturated fat content of coconut oil. This is because as well as containing saturated fat, coconut oil is also high in lauric acid, which is a kind of fat that is rarely found in nature. When lauric acid enters the body it is converted into monolaurin, which has powerful antiviral and antibacterial qualities. Additionally, the medium-chain fatty acids that are abundant in coconut oil are perfect for promoting optimum health in the body. They have shown great potential in protecting against diabetes and heart disease.

If you lead a fairly sedentary lifestyle then it is all the more important to avoid saturated fat. The combination of inactivity and poor food choices makes your chance of ill health all the more prevalent. At best I would suggest that the amount of fat you consume should only be 10–20 percent of the total calories you eat in a day. If a small portion of this percentage comes from saturated fat then that is not something to worry too much about.

The foods highest in saturated fat are meat, dairy products made with whole milk, and processed snack foods. It is also commonly found in commercially manufactured baked goods.

Monounsaturated fat

Monounsaturated fat is found in abundance in nuts and certain plant oils. Monounsaturated fats have a single carbon-to-carbon double bond. This basically means that it has fewer hydrogen atoms than saturated fat.

In contrast to trans and saturated fat, monounsaturated fat is good for you and can help to lower LDL cholesterol levels, Monounsaturated fat is also thought to be good for regulating insulin levels in the body and controlling blood sugar levels.

The best sources of monounsaturated fat are avocados, many different kinds of nuts, and olive oil. Aiming to include at least one of these things in your diet every day will go a long way to protecting your health.

Polyunsaturated fat

Found mostly in plant-based foods and oils, polyunsaturated fats, similar to monounsaturated fat, is beneficial to health, especially in relation to lowering LDL cholesterol levels and protecting your cardiovascular system. Research has suggested that polyunsaturated fats are of particular use in preventing the onset of type 2 diabetes.[6,7]

Polyunsaturated fats are essential fats, which means they are absolutely necessary in the body for it to continue functioning as normal. However, your body is unable to make this kind of fat on its own, so it's important to get it from dietary sources. The uses of polyunsaturated fat in the body range from reducing inflammation to helping the blood clot properly, as well as building strong cell membranes and enabling optimum muscle movement. There is also early research to suggest that polyunsaturated fat could be useful in lowering risk factors associated with dementia.[8]

The best plant-based sources of polyunsaturated fats are nuts (especially walnuts), and flaxseeds.

A peek at avocados and why you'll want to eat them

Just one serving of avocado will provide your body with approximately 20 different vitamins and minerals. This includes healthy doses of potassium, lutein, and folate, as well as an abundance of vitamins C, E, and a range of B vitamins. They are low in sugar but high in fiber, which, as we know, means they can help you to feel full for longer. Avocados are also completely free from cholesterol and sodium.

The impressive nutrient count aside, avocados are also high in monounsaturated fat, which, as we covered earlier, is a good fat. In fact, more than 50 percent of the total fat count of this fruit is of the monounsaturated variety. When we consider that avocado is one of the only fruits that contains monounsaturated fat, then the high levels found within are even more impressive! They also contain polyunsaturated fat, albeit in a smaller amount than the monounsaturated variety.

Often when we buy avocados they will not have ripened fully and will need to be left for a few days. You can speed up the ripening process by storing them with a banana or an apple. This is because bananas and apples release a gas called ethylene, a hormone that triggers ripening.

A peek at nuts and why you'll want to eat them

Nuts frequently get a bad rap for being so high in fat but when we look at the kind of fats they contain, they don't look so bad after all!

As well as containing heart healthy fats, nuts are also rich in protein, fiber, and a wide range of vitamins and minerals.

However, there are still a few things that you need to consider when snacking on nuts. First of all, as with most things, moderation is key. Even though they contain high levels of beneficial fats, they are also high in calories. Second, always choose the raw, unsalted variety, as this is the best way to get the benefits of nuts without the unhealthy aspects.

So which nuts should you be stocking your cupboards with?

Walnuts

Walnuts are the most antioxidant rich of all the nuts. They are amazing for protecting the body from damage to cells, which in turn helps to protect you against cancer, heart disease, and age-related diseases. They are also a fantastic source of omega-3 fatty acids, which are essential for fighting inflammation. Omega-3 fatty acids fall into the unsaturated category and are found most predominantly in fish. So, if you're following a plant-based diet then eating these nuts will help to keep a deficiency at bay. Walnuts are a particularly good choice for women as the high manganese count can help to relieve PMS symptoms.

One serving of 7 walnuts = 185 calories and 18g fat

Almonds

Almonds are absolutely crammed full of fiber and contain the most vitamin E of all the nuts. Research has shown that almonds are beneficial to those who are trying to lose weight or manage their blood sugar.[9,10] Eating a serving every day can help to lower LDL cholesterol levels and insulin resistance. These amazing little nuts have also been shown to increase the presence of good bacteria in the body, which gives your immune system a boost! The majority of fat in almonds is the monounsaturated type with a dose of polyunsaturated included, too.

One serving of 20 nuts = 139 calories and 12g fat

Cashew nuts

Cashew nuts are favored for their high iron and zinc count, but they are also a great source of magnesium. This means by eating them regularly you will supply your body with iron: essential for delivering oxygen to your cells; zinc which boosts your immune system and vision; and magnesium, which is great for your memory! Cashew nuts are rich in monounsaturated fat and several phytochemicals that are great for all-round health.

One serving of 18 nuts = 165 calories and 13g fat

Pecans

Pecans contain high levels of monounsaturated fat and also favorable amounts of polyunsaturated fat. There is also a small natural presence of saturated fat. Studies have shown that they are amazing artery defenders, which can help to combat plaque formation inside the arteries. Research has also shown them to be beneficial for brain health as the high presence of antioxidants can combat the progression of age related degenerative diseases.[11]

One serving of 9 nuts = 200 calories and 21g fat

Brazil nuts

Eating just one Brazil nut every day will ensure you hit your recommended dose of selenium for the day. Selenium has powerful antioxidant qualities that have been linked to lower rates of certain cancers, such as breast cancer, prostate cancer, and bone cancer. Brazil nuts are high in calories but the majority of the fat is of the monounsaturated variety.

One serving of 6 nuts = 186 calories and 18g fat

Pistachios

Raw, unsalted pistachios only pack approximately four calories in each nut! Having to shell them before you eat them has also been shown to lead to a lower consumption than other types of nuts. This generally leads to fewer calories consumed, making pistachios great for those looking for a weight loss snack. Only a small portion of the fat in pistachios is saturated and the rest is a healthy combination of monounsaturated and polyunsaturated fat.

These great little nuts are a serious source of potassium and fibre. Approximately 50 contain as much potassium as an orange and the same fibre as half a cup of broccoli. FDA research suggests that eating an adequate amount of nuts every day can help to reduce heart disease risk, so there's no reason not to indulge on this snack!

One serving of 25 nuts = 80 calories and 7g fat

A peek at seeds and why you'll want to eat them

People often dismiss seeds as a food source because they are not commonly seen as a tasty option. However, many varieties of seeds in their raw form are actually quite delicious. And, what's more, they are also incredibly nutritious! As well as containing an exciting range of vitamins and minerals, seeds also pack a high count of phytosterols that are great for lowering LDL cholesterol levels! So which seeds should you have stored in your kitchen?

Sunflower seeds

As well as producing beautiful flowers, sunflower seeds are also a plentiful source of health-boosting nutrients. When eaten raw they have a nutty taste and crunchy consistency, and they make a great addition to cereals, salads, and rice dishes.

Sunflower seeds are a great source of selenium, calcium, copper, magnesium, and vitamin E. As I mentioned above, selenium is useful for cancer prevention and calcium, copper, and magnesium all play a role in keeping our bones strong. Vitamin E has many uses, not least the protection it provides for your skin against harmful UV rays.

117

Sunflower seeds have powerful anti-inflammatory properties, which means they are useful for relieving a wide range of conditions, such as arthritis and pain in the joints.

If you are looking for a way to boost your energy throughout the day, then a handful of sunflower seeds could be the answer. They are high in calories at approximately 580 calories per 100g but the majority of these calories come from polyunsaturated fatty acids. They also contain an ample amount of monounsaturated fat. When consumed regularly the beneficial fats in sunflower seeds can help to prevent bad cholesterol from collecting in the arteries.

⅛ cup/18.5g of sunflower seeds = 84 calories and 7.5g fat

Pumpkin seeds

Pumpkin seeds are similar to sunflower seeds in that they contain impressive amounts of health boosting nutrients. In fact, just one serving (¼ cup/32g) will provide approximately half your daily recommended dose of magnesium. This serving also packs a powerful punch of zinc, which many people struggle to consume an adequate amount of, and of particular benefit to men due to the role of zinc in prostate health.

Early research shows that pumpkin seeds may be of use in regulating insulin production due their ability to reduce oxidative stress in the body, which means good things for diabetics.[12,13] Women who are postmenopausal can also benefit from pumpkin seeds because of the wealth of phytoestrogens they contain. Studies have shown that these phytoestrogens increase HDL cholesterol, lower blood pressure, and also relieve hot flashes (flushes), and other symptoms associated with menopause.[14,15]

Eating pumpkin seeds that still have the kernel is the best option for heart health, as the kernel contains particularly high levels of monounsaturated fat. It is always best to eat them raw and if possible choose the organic version to avoid any potentially harmful contaminants.

¼ cup/32g of pumpkin seeds = 71 calories and 3g fat

Hemp seeds

Hemp plants are among the most nutritious in the world and the seeds are also an amazing source of nutrition. They provide a complete protein as they contain all nine of the essential amino acids, as well as a great range of minerals, vitamins, and essential fats. Hemp seeds are especially rich in vitamin E as well as potassium, fiber, iron, and magnesium. Just two tablespoons of hemp seeds will provide you with an impressive 2g of fiber and 5g of protein. Going the extra mile and including three tablespoons in your diet every day will mean you instantly hit 50 percent of your recommended daily allowance of magnesium and phosphorous. This amount also contains 25 percent of your recommended daily allowance of zinc and 15 percent for iron. They are also free from saturated fats, starch, and sugar making them all the better for our health!

Hemp seeds have been cultivated for many thousands of years and consumed in their whole form. These seeds can be used to create several other nutritional products such as hemp flour or hemp milk. However, it is also possible (but less common) to use the seeds to make hemp oil and protein powder, but you will find more and more energy bars and cereals that include hemp seeds.

Regularly eating hemp seeds is thought to aid weight loss, promote better energy, lower LDL cholesterol levels, boost the immune system, and also improve your circulation. It is also believed that hemp seeds can be used as a powerful way to manage your blood sugar levels.

Many of the fatty acids found in hemp seeds are a combination of both omega-3s and omega-6s. In fact, up to 80 percent of these fatty acids are of the polyunsaturated variety, making them great for heart health. There is also a slight presence of monounsaturated fats for an extra boost.

The seeds have quite a nutty flavor and make a tasty addition to many dishes. I believe they go best with granola, soup, or salad. In order to maintain maximum nutritional value I recommend that you eat them raw but that doesn't mean you can't also benefit from using them in baking or cooking if you wish to.

¼ cup/7.5g of hemp seeds = 180 calories and 15g fat

Flaxseeds

Flaxseeds are impressively high in omega-3 fatty acid and are considered to be one of the best sources of this heart-healthy fat. The most prevalent omega-3 fatty acid in these amazing seeds is known as alpha-linolenic acid. This particular acid is known to be essential in preventing inflammation in the cardiovascular system, promoting optimum function. The presence of omega-3 fatty acids means that these seeds are of use to people who are trying to lower their blood pressure. Early studies have shown them to be of some benefit for people suffering with hypertension.[16] Statistics show that approximately one in three people have high blood pressure. Although there is medication available to control this, it is also possible to achieve lower blood pressure through your dietary choices.

Another impressive fact about these little seeds is that they contain fiber-like compounds known as lignans. These offer some of the same benefits of fiber but also boast antioxidant properties that, as we know, will help to battle those free radicals in your body. Studies have shown that flaxseeds are the best natural source of lignans and that regularly including this food in your diet is fantastic for overall health.[17]

Another interesting fact about flaxseeds is that they contain a water-soluble, gel-forming substance that boosts the function of the intestinal tract. When this substance is present, the stomach takes longer to pass food to the small intestine, so there is more opportunity for the small intestine to absorb the nutrients it needs.

The anti-inflammatory and antioxidant benefits of flaxseeds are not only great for cardiovascular health but also for preventing certain other health problems. Regular consumption can help to prevent insulin resistance, diabetes, and obesity. There is also evidence to suggest these seeds could be useful in preventing cancer because of their ability to limit oxidative stress. Studies that have been conducted into this potential have shown that they could be of most benefit in preventing colon cancer, prostate cancer and breast cancer.[18-20]

Your digestive tract has much to gain when you consume flaxseeds; they are high in fiber-like compounds, lignans, so contribute to the steady movement of food through the digestive system.

Flaxseeds can be purchased in a range of colors, most usually they will be a variety of yellow shades to brown or red colors. It is also possible to find green or white flaxseeds, but these colors indicate that they have been harvested before they were ready. On the other hand, black flaxseeds have not been harvested in time. When consuming flaxseeds for their high nutritional count, I would recommend avoiding the green, white and black varieties.

Like the other seeds discussed in this section, flaxseeds have also been shown to be useful in lowering LDL cholesterol.

¼ cup/37.5g of flaxseeds = 224 calories and 18g fat

Seven simple recipes that include good fats

Here are seven great-tasting recipes to get you going on your journey to incorporating healthy fats into your diet every day.

Apple and Avocado Smoothie

A great smoothie for a quick breakfast or for an energizing snack, this smoothie rocks!

Serves 1

½ avocado, peeled and destoned

1 green apple, roughly chopped

1 cup/8fl oz/225ml coconut milk

1 cup/2½oz/70g spinach

Juice ½ lemon

3 ice cubes

Place all the ingredients in a blender and blitz until smooth. When blending with ice it is best to start on a low speed and gradually speed up. Alternatively you can blitz it first and serve over ice.

Chickpea and Avocado Salad

This light and tasty salad is packed with lashings of good fats and fiber, making it the perfect lunchtime dish.

Serves 2

- 1 head of Romaine lettuce, roughly shredded
- Handful fresh cilantro (coriander), trimmed and chopped
- 1 medium tomato, diced
- 1 red bell pepper, deseeded and finely sliced
- 14 oz/400g can chickpeas, drained and rinsed
- 1 tbsp lemon juice
- 2 tbsp flaxseeds
- Pinch of pink Himalayan sea salt
- Pinch of freshly ground black pepper
- 1 large ripe avocado, peeled, destoned and chopped into large chunks

Place the Romaine and cilantro (coriander) in a large salad bowl then add the tomato and red pepper. Toss gently with your hands to combine.

In a separate bowl toss the chickpeas in the lemon juice, flaxseeds, sea salt and pepper. Give a quick stir to make sure the flavor is spread evenly and then add the chickpeas to the salad bowl, too.

The final step is to add the avocado to the salad bowl before serving immediately.

Homemade Cashew Nut Butter

A delicious alternative to dairy butter that is easy to make and much more nutritious!

Makes approximately 1½ cups/13 oz/375g

3 cups/1 lb/450g raw cashew nuts

1 tbsp raw honey

1 tbsp coconut oil

Soak the cashew nuts by placing them in a bowl and covering with water and leaving for 3–4 hours.

Drain and rinse the cashews before placing them in a blender with the honey and coconut oil. Start on a slow speed and then work your way up to a high speed. It will take some time for the cashew nuts to blend completely into butter. Feel free to give your blender a bit of a break at regular intervals, and give the mixture a stir to make sure it is not clumping. The entire process of blending the cashew nuts can take 15–30 minutes, so be patient!

When the butter has a smooth consistency, place in an airtight container and store in your refrigerator, where it will keep fresh for up to two weeks.

Mixed Nut Burgers

Not keen on veggie burgers? Well, I urge you to give this recipe a try! Top with your favorite relish, pickles, onions, tomatoes, or mustard and enjoy!

Makes 6 burgers

1 cup/8oz/225g bulgur wheat, uncooked

⅓ cup/1¾oz/50g raw cashew nuts, finely chopped

⅓ cup/1¾oz/50g raw almonds, finely chopped

⅓ cup/1¾oz/50g raw Brazil nuts, finely chopped

2 tbsp ground flaxseeds

6 tbsp water

1 tbsp coconut oil plus extra for cooking

1 tbsp whole wheat (all-purpose) flour

½ tsp ground cumin

First, bring a large pan of water to the boil and cook the bulgur wheat for 10 minutes, or according to packet instructions. Drain any excess water and set aside to cool.

Place the cashew nuts, almonds and Brazil nuts into a large bowl. (To ensure that the nuts are finely chopped, you might want to give them a quick blitz in your blender or food processor.)

Add the ground flaxseed, water, coconut oil, flour, and cumin. Stir well to ensure that all the ingredients are combined. Once the bulgur wheat is cooled to room temperature, add it to the bowl and stir well to combine.

Divide the mixture into six equal parts then form your burgers by rolling into balls and gently flattening with the heel of your hand.

Drizzle a little coconut oil into a large skillet (frying pan) and leave to heat for a couple of minutes. When the oil if hot, add the burgers and fry for 5 minutes each side.

Serve in whole-wheat buns or with your favorite salad dish.

Pumpkin Seed Cookies

If you like banana bread, then you'll love these cookies that use bananas instead of eggs—a great substitution if you're avoiding animal products. Combine that with the pumpkin seeds, and you have a yummy snack at your fingertips.

Makes 8 good-sized cookies

2 ripe bananas, peeled and chopped

½ cup/1½ oz/40g coconut palm sugar

2 tbsp coconut oil

2 cups/10oz/300g whole wheat (all-purpose) flour, sifted

1 cup/5oz/140g pumpkin seeds

¼ cup/1¼oz/35g cashew nuts, chopped

½ tbsp baking powder, sifted

½ tsp baking soda (bicarbonate of soda), sifted

Preheat the oven to 425°F/220°C/gas mark 7 and grease a non-stick cookie tray with a little coconut oil.

Place the bananas in a bowl with the coconut palm sugar and coconut oil and stir until thoroughly mixed.

Next add the flour, pumpkin seeds, cashew nuts, baking powder, and baking soda (bicarbonate of soda) to the bowl and mix well until combined.

Form the dough into balls about the size of golf ball and place on the cookie tray. Gently flatten each of the balls to create your cookies. Make sure you leave at least 2in (5cm) between each cookie so they have space to expand in the oven.

Place in a preheated oven for approximately 10 minutes or until the edges turn a golden brown color.

These cookies will stay fresh in an airtight container for three days.

Hemp Seed Smoothie Bowl

Think of this as almost like a chocolate milkshake but filled with all things good! Impossible you might think... But give this one a go and I think you'll agree it's thick, creamy, and slightly chocolatey, too!

Serves 2

2 cups/5oz/140g spinach

2 cups/5oz/140g kale

½ cucumber, roughly chopped

1 ripe banana

½ avocado, peeled and destoned

1 tbsp hemp seeds

1 tsp spirulina

1 cup/8fl oz/225ml coconut milk

1 tbsp raw cacao

A handful of ice (optional)

Place all the ingredients except the ice in a blender and blitz for about 2 minutes or until thick and creamy.

If you want to chill the smoothie, add the ice to the blender and blitz again.

Spoon into bowls and serve immediately.

Creamy Butternut Squash Soup

This is quite possibly my favorite soup of all time—super creamy, super filling, and super delicious.

Serves 2-3

4 tbsp coconut oil

1 large onion

2 cloves garlic, peeled and minced

1in (2.5cm) fresh root ginger

1 cup/5½oz/150g raw cashew nuts

1 butternut squash, peeled, deseeded and chopped into 1in (2.5cm) chunks

2 carrots, peeled and diced

4 cups/1½ pints/900ml vegetable stock

1 tsp ground cumin

1 tsp ground turmeric

Pinch of pink Himalayan sea salt

Pinch of freshly ground black pepper

2-3 handfuls of fresh cilantro (coriander), trimmed and chopped.

Place the coconut oil in a large pan on a medium heat to warm for a couple of minutes. Add the onion, garlic, and ginger, and sauté for about 4–5 minutes. Next add the cashew nuts and continue to cook for a further 4–5 minutes.

Add the butternut squash, carrots, vegetable stock, cumin and turmeric to the pan and stir well to combine. Reduce the heat and leave to simmer for 25–30 minutes. Then use a hand blender or food processor to blitz the soup to a smooth liquid.

Return the soup to the pan, on a medium-heat, and season with sea salt and pepper to taste. Stir well and leave to cook for a further 3–5 minutes.

Ladle into bowls and garnish each with fresh cilantro (coriander) before serving.

Chapter 6

Get the "Super" Back into Your Diet

Learn how and why to include goji berries, chia seeds, spirulina, bee pollen, and cacao easily and effortlessly in your diet every day.

This is quite possibly one of my favorite subjects! It seems as if every day there is new study or claim that comes out championing the extraordinary super powers of superfoods. I like to think of them as a class of their own, providing maximum nutrition and packed with health!

So what do superfoods do for your body and health?

Superfoods can significantly improve our overall health by increasing energy, boosting the immune system, cleansing the body, and exceeding our protein, vitamin, mineral, and essential fatty acid requirements. As a bonus, superfoods rid us of the need to take endless supplements. If you're ridding your body of packaged and process foods and eating a whole-food, varied diet, you'll get all the nutrition you need from those whole foods. Thank goodness! Simply put, superfoods are a guaranteed way to get a super highway of nutrients moving through your body in a super spectacular way.

Superfoods strengthen your immune system

A strong immune system is essential, if we are to keep things like viruses and infections at bay, and it needs constant nourishment in order to function at its optimum level. There are, of course, things we can do to protect ourselves from germs and bacteria, such as keeping good personal hygiene, however, the food we eat also plays a huge part in protecting us from external influences that can threaten our health.

Rather than taking supplements, which are not made naturally and often don't contain the nutrients you need in the right amounts, you can eat a few tasty superfoods and get optimum levels of the same nutrients. This means your body will have everything it needs to fight off illnesses and keep you functioning at its best.

Superfoods fight free radicals

Free radicals are atoms that have degraded in some way and can damage cells in the body by putting other atoms into an imbalance. Superfoods, however, contain antioxidants that neutralize free radicals by replacing the parts of the atoms that free radicals steal, which mean they can effectively stop the damage being caused. When we eat foods that have a high antioxidant count, we are equipping our bodies to combat free radicals, which in turn means less damage is done to our cells.

Superfoods can reduce the risk of cancer

Studies by leading cancer research organizations[1-3] have shown that eating a wide range of highly concentrated plant foods—such as superfoods—can increase our protection against cancer-causing agents—such as free radicals and carcinogens.

In addition, studies have shown that superfoods can be of use to those suffering with cancer because it is essential that cancer patients maintain a strong immune system to aid their eventual recovery,[4,5] and that's exactly where superfoods come in. Treatments for cancer can be incredibly damaging to the body, and a diet full of immunity-boosting superfoods during this time can help restore the body's normal functions.

We also know from this research that while no one food will be enough to provide the comprehensive range of nutrients your body needs to remain at optimum health, superfoods do have largely beneficial health-boosting properties due to their high levels of antioxidants, vitamins, and minerals.

Superfoods can help to keep your heart healthy

As I mentioned in a previous chapter (*see page 33*), heart disease is responsible for more than 25 percent of all deaths in the USA today.[6] When we consider that research shows that a healthy, varied diet and regular exercise is a great way to help prevent disease, it is astonishing that the figures are still so high.[7]

Superfoods play a huge role in preserving the health of your heart and, again, this is largely due the high presence of antioxidants inside them.

One particular type of antioxidant called a flavonoid, which is found in raw cacao, has been shown in studies to help dilate, or increase, the blood vessels, which in turn helps to decrease blood pressure and improve circulation—both of which lead to better heart health.[8,9]

Superfoods increase your energy

With busy lives and the constant demands that go hand in hand with trying to strike a work-family balance, we can find that our energy levels need a boost to get us through the day. When this happens, most people tend to rely on coffee and other stimulants to help them cope. This is of course a dangerous path to take, as dependency and addiction can easily begin to cause greater problems to our health.

The food that we consume greatly influences our energy levels, and it is important to understand what our bodies need. Really getting to grips with the different nutrients our bodies require and where you can find them will help you to understand what things you should be eating in order to maximize your health. It will also importantly help you to understand why you should be eating them.

Protein is useful for improving overall brain function and increasing alertness and performance, making it an essential in our diet. It is the basic building block for generating hormones, enzymes, and cells. Two of the superfoods I recommend, goji berries and spirulina, are especially high in protein.

Fiber helps to stabilize blood sugar and the amount of insulin we produce, which means that our energy levels are much more likely to be steady, as opposed to flucluating dramatically throughout the day. Fibrous superfoods include cacao, one of my recommended superfoods. If consumed in powder form, just two tablespoons of cacao a day will give you about 3.5g of the all-important dietary fiber.

Fatty acids, such as omega-3 and omega-6, are great for maintaining a strong heart and keeping hormone levels in balance. Chia seeds, the all-round superfood hero, have fatty acids aplenty among a host of other great nutrients.

Superfoods boost your metabolism

When we eat food, hormones are produced inside our bodies. Some of these hormones are responsible for stimulating our metabolism to burn more fat, whereas others slow the metabolism down. Therefore, the foods that you choose to eat can have a direct impact on the productivity of your metabolism.

Superfoods are naturally produced plant-based foods and, as a result, have a positive effect on your metabolism. Containing high levels of vitamins for a better metabolic function, and full of healthy nutrients, such as protein and fiber, superfoods can help your body to burn the energy sources it should be burning (i.e. fatty deposits).

Superfoods can help keep you young

When it comes to the youthful appearance of our skin, there is nothing better than getting the antioxidants from superfoods into our diet. Studies have shown that they can protect against premature aging of the skin. Vitamin E is the most commonly referenced antioxidant when it comes to skin health, and several superfoods contain high levels of this nutrient.[10]

Free radicals, as described earlier, are known to cause damage to cells in general, but more specifically, they damage collagen and dehydrate the skin. They can even be responsible for the premature occurrence of wrinkles. However, when antioxidants are present in abundance in the body, they work to neutralize these free radicals and to prevent these signs of premature aging. Regularly consuming superfoods keeps your levels of antioxidants high and can keep you looking younger.

A peek at goji berries and why you'll want to eat them

Goji berries are one of the most nutritious foods on the planet. They are native to China, Tibet, and Mongolia but they are now also grown in other parts of the world. In the grand scheme of things, they are still a relatively new food in the West, but that hasn't stopped many people discovering, enjoying, and benefiting from them!

Goji berries naturally contain everything the human body needs to be healthy because they contain all the necessary amino acids, which is incredibly rare. They also have a very high protein count for a fruit. Goji berries boast high levels of vitamin C and fiber, as well as having more carotenoids than any other food. Carotenoids are the reason why fruits and vegetables can have such a strong color, but they also have health benefits. Additionally, a significant amount of iron, calcium, zinc, and selenium can be found in a single serving of these berries.

As well as being a powerhouse for nutrition, goji berries also contain antifungal, antibacterial, and anti-inflammatory properties, making them a staple of Traditional Chinese Medicine (TCM). The Chinese have long believed that goji berries increase strength and longevity, and evidently science is beginning to prove that as well.[11]

Goji berries are most commonly available in a dried form, which makes them perfect to munch on as a snack. You can also easily add them into cereal or smoothies to instantly increase the nutritional value of your meal.

A peek at chia seeds and why you'll want to eat them

These little seeds are absolutely loaded with nutrients that are great for both body and mind. They are cultivated from the *Salvia Hispanica* plant native to South America. "Chia" is the Mayan word for strength, and the ancient Mayan and Aztec civilizations prized these seeds for being a valuable source of sustainable energy. Naturally free from gluten, chia seeds are also usually grown organically, making them ideal for allergy-sufferers or those looking to keep their food as close to nature as possible.

The popularity of the chia seed has truly exploded over the past few years but with very good reason! A single 28g serving packs an impressive 11g of fiber and 4g of protein. The same 28g serving will also provide you with 30 percent of your recommended daily dose of manganese—which helps keeps bones strong—and magnesium—which helps the body create and maintain enzyme production. It also provides 27 percent of your recommended daily dose of phosphorus, which, like manganese, helps with bone strength and is the second most common mineral found in the human body.

Chia seeds contain large amounts of antioxidants, which protect the essential fats in the seed from becoming rancid. These are mostly omega-3 fatty acids, which are known to be great for many aspects of your health, not least of all for protecting your heart.

If that wasn't enough to make you rush to nearest health food store and stock up, Chia seeds are widely acknowledged to be an excellent weight-loss tool due to their high fiber and protein count. When chia seeds enter your stomach they absorb water and expand, which helps you to feel fuller for longer.

A peek at spirulina and why you'll want to eat it

An algae that grows on fresh, warm water, spirulina has been cultivated for many thousands of years. It grows comfortably even in the harshest of conditions, which has led many experts to question its potential in their quest to end world hunger.[12] Studies have confirmed its medicinal use in treating a range of ailments, such as candida overgrowth and even arsenic poisoning.[13]

Spirulina has one of the highest levels of protein found in any edible substance. Just 10g of this superfood will yield 6g of protein, which is 13 percent of the RDA for women and just over 11 percent for men,[14] making it ideal for encouraging your body to heal and repair.

Just adding 2g of spirulina to your diet every day can help boost your immune system and stabilize your blood pressure. It can even help you to get your cholesterol under control by lowering your LDL cholesterol levels.

A peek at bee pollen and why you'll want to eat it

It is important to distinguish between bee pollen and honey because they are two very different things. We looked at the benefits of honey in a previous chapter (*see page 73*) but bee pollen is the substance that worker bees pack into pellets to be made into honey, and it is incredibly nourishing for both bees and humans.

In fact, bee pollen contains almost all of the nutrients that people need. It takes one bee working eight hours a day for a month to make just one teaspoon of bee pollen, so it is very precious. Bee pollen is crammed full of vitamins and minerals, as well as carbohydrates, lipids, and proteins, all of which are necessary for a healthily functioning body.

Studies have determined the efficiency of bee pollen in slowing down or preventing the growth of bacteria due to its antibacterial properties.[15,16] The same studies also show that regular consumption of bee pollen can help people with a low red blood cell count, as it helps the presence of these cells to grow considerably.

The potential to treat allergies is one of the most exciting health aspects of studies of bee pollen, and it seems that when allergy-sufferers consume this superfood, it stimulates their immune system to produce additional antibodies that work to prevent allergic reactions.[17]

Research has also shown that bee pollen could be effective for those wishing to lose weight.[18,19] This is because it works to boost the metabolism thereby increasing your body's effectiveness in burning calories.

Including bee pollen in your diet every day can really help to get your skin looking its best as well. This is due, in large part, to the fact that it works to protect us against dehydration—a prime cause of dull-looking skin.

A peek at cacao and why you'll want to eat it

Cacao, when eaten in its raw form, is incredibly good for you. Raw cacao is made by cold-pressing non-roasted cocoa beans, which allows the living enzymes to remain inside while removing the fat. When cacao is processed through roasting, instead of cold pressing, the end product is cocoa powder, which is nowhere near as nutritious as the original seed.

Studies have shown that regular consumption of raw cacao protects the nervous system, reduces the risk of stroke, lowers blood pressure, helps to protect the heart, and also helps to protect cells from damage.[20,21] It is also useful in lowering insulin resistance. As described in a previous chapter, insulin resistance is a precursor to type 2 diabetes and other insulin-related illnesses (*see page 66*), so it is important to keep this resistance at a low level.

Many of these great health benefits exist because raw cacao is a powerhouse of antioxidants, and also loaded with minerals, including manganese, copper, potassium, calcium, zinc, iron, and magnesium. Copper is a trace mineral that is incredibly important for the body to be healthy, and is found in the liver, heart, kidneys, brain, and muscles. It also helps to make collagen, so helps keep your looking young. Calcium is well known for its relationship with healthy bones, and iron metabolizes the proteins in your blood, a necessary function for survival.

Seven recipes that include superfoods

Here are seven of my favourite recipes to get you going on your journey to incorporating superfoods effortlessly into your diet every day.

Superfood Smoothie

Here you have two of the superfoods in one super smoothie. But don't forget that just like goji berries and cacao, you have a few other super foods in this one too, such as kale, blueberries, and even lucuma.

Serves 1–2

> 1 tbsp goji berries
>
> 2 cups/16fl oz/450ml coconut water
>
> 1 banana, peeled
>
> 1 tsp lucuma powder
>
> 1 tsp raw cacao
>
> ½ cup/2oz/55g blueberries
>
> Handful of kale

Presoak the goji berries in a bowl of cold water for 10 minutes before draining and rinsing.

Place the berries in a blender with the rest of the ingredients and blitz for 1–2 minutes or until smooth.

Serve immediately.

Chia Seed Cookies

This recipe is jam packed with chia seeds—literally! If you're looking for a way to get your family to eat more superfoods, then this recipe is a great place to start. The coconut sugar also means it's super sweet so a real treat for anyone with a sweet tooth.

Makes 8 cookies

> ½ cup/1½oz/40g coconut palm sugar
>
> ½ cup/6oz/175g organic runny honey
>
> 1 tsp vanilla extract
>
> ½ cup/2½oz/75g whole wheat (all-purpose) flour, sifted

¼ tsp baking powder, sifted

1 tbsp chia seeds

3 tbsp water

Preheat the oven to 400°F/200°C/gas mark 6 and grease a cookie tray with a little coconut oil.

Place the coconut palm sugar, honey, vanilla extract, flour, and baking powder together in a bowl. Stir well to combine and form a sticky dough.

Once this is combined well slowly add the chia seeds and water to the mixture, stirring well in between to combine!

Shape the dough into golf-ball-size balls, place on the cookie tray, leaving at least 2in (5cm) between each cookie so they have space to expand in the oven, and then gently flatten each of the balls to form the cookies.

Place in a preheated oven and bake for approximately 10 minutes until golden. Remove from the oven and leave to cool on a wire rack.

Eat immediately or store in airtight container for up to three days

Creamy Super Soup

A super simple way to eat spirulina without having to taste it! If you're a fan of raw foods then just skip heating the soup—it tastes great either way.

Serves 2

2 cups raw cashew nuts

2 cups/16fl oz/450ml water or vegetable stock

2 cups/5oz/140g kale

2 cups/5oz/140g spinach

1 avocado, peeled and destoned

A handful of fresh cilantro (coriander), trimmed

1in (2.5cm) fresh root ginger, peeled

2 cloves of garlic, peeled

1 tbsp spirulina

1 tsp cumin

Place the cashew nuts and water into your blender and blitz for about 5 minutes or until smooth.

Next add the rest of the ingredients to the blender and continue to blend until everything is completely smooth about 1–2 minutes.

Pour the soup into a medium saucepan and heat on a low heat for 10–15 minutes.

Divide into bowl and serve immediately.

Green Glow Salad Dressing

I'm always looking for a killer salad dressing and this one hits the mark. It's also an easy way to incorporate that vitamin-packed bee pollen into your diet too. No one will know either!

Serves 4

½ an avocado, peeled and destoned

Juice of 1 lemon

A handful of fresh mint

4 tbsp flaxseed oil

2 tsp bee pollen

Place all the ingredients in a blender and blitz to a smooth, runny consistency.

Drizzle over your favorite salad for a superfood boost.

Raw Cacao Bars

Filled with amazing nuts, natural sweeteners and the added bonus of chocolate, these bars are sure to give you a good boost of healthy energy!

Makes 10 bars

2 cups/6oz/175g oats

1 cup/6oz/175g dates

3 tbsp raw cacao

½ cup/2½oz/70g raw cashew nuts

1 tbsp pumpkin seeds

½ cup/4oz/115g almond butter

½ cup/1½ oz/40g coconut palm sugar

2 tbsp organic runny honey

2 tbsp water

Place 1 cup of the oats in a bowl and cover the oats with cold water so that they are just submerged. Leave to soak for 30 minutes before transferring them to a blender.

Add the dates, raw cacao, and cashew nuts to the blender with another cup of oats, the pumpkin seeds, almond butter, coconut palm sugar, honey, and water; blitz to create a smooth consistency.

Transfer the mixture to a large bowl and use your hands to knead the mixture for about 2 minutes until it forms a soft dough.

Place the dough in a 8×8 (20×20) bake pan (cake tin) lined with parchment paper and flatten with the back of spoon to an equal depth across the bake pan. Place in the refrigerator for 2 hours until firm. Cut into 10 small bars and serve.

Chia Seed Loaf

Looking to make something completely different but utterly good for you? Then this loaf has your name on it, and also makes an amazing addition to any dinner party.

Makes 1 loaf

1 cup/5oz/150g whole wheat (all-purpose) flour
⅔ cup/6oz/175g soy or coconut yogurt
1½ tsp baking powder
1 tsp baking soda
½ cup/5½oz/150g coconut oil
½ cup/1½oz/40g coconut palm sugar
2 tbsp ground flax seeds

6 tbsp water

1oz/30g chia seeds

Juice of 1 lemon

Handful of raisins (optional)

Preheat the oven to 350°C/180°F/gas mark 4 and line a 1lb (450g) bread pan (bread tin) with baking parchment.

Place the flour, yogurt, baking powder and baking soda (bicarbonate of soda) in a bowl and whisk until well combined.

In a separate bowl mix the coconut oil and the coconut palm sugar together 3–4 minutes until combined.

In another bowl mix the ground flax seeds and water before adding to the coconut oil and sugar. Next add the lemon zest and chia seeds (and raisins, if you like) into this bowl too and mix well.

Finally pour this mixture over the flour, yogurt, baking powder, and baking soda (bicarbonate of soda), and mix well to form a smooth batter before pouring into your prepared bread pan. Bake in a preheated oven for 45 minutes until golden. After this time, remove the loaf from the oven and leave to cool for a few minutes before turning it out of the bread pan (bread tin).

Cut into slices and serve with some nut butter and a drizzle of honey. Stored in a cool dark place, this loaf will keep fresh for up to three days.

Goji Berry Ice Cream

Making ice cream doesn't always require an ice-cream maker, and this healthier version makes a delicious treat on a hot summer's day.

Serves 4

½ cup/2oz/55g goji berries

1 ripe banana, peeled and frozen

½ cup/2oz/55g frozen blueberries

½ cup/3oz/85g pitted dates

1 tsp ground cinnamon

Presoak the goji berries in a bowl of cold water for 10 minutes before rinsing and draining.

Place the berries in a blender with the rest of the ingredients and blitz for about 2 minutes or until the mixture forms a smooth creamy consistency.

Spoon the mixture into an airtight container and freeze for 3–4 hours until frozen. Serve with fresh fruit or alone for a deliciously simple treat.

Chapter 7

Five Simple Rules on Eating Out

Learn how and why to eat well while dining out with my five simple tricks.

I'm constantly on the go... whether that's chauffeuring my four kids around, teaching yoga, or cycling to get to a meeting... My days are pretty jam packed and I often get asked, "How do you eat healthily when you're not in your own kitchen—especially when you're out to lunch and dinner?" Just because you want to eat a healthy diet doesn't mean you have to become a social bore! I'm such an 80/20 kinda gal. It is the approach that works best for me. I eat well and clean 80 percent of the time and then the other 20 percent I eat foods that might not be 100 percent clean, but only in moderation. It's important not to stress about eating out as that can wreak more havoc on your body than the "unhealthy" meal you might have to eat.

Remember this: It's your journey, your adventure, your body, and your right to eating healthily! As with anything in life, it just takes time. So stay resilient in your path. Trust me, you will never ever regret it.

Rule 1: Keep it real

There is absolutely always going to be something healthy on the menu wherever you are dining out. The majority of places that serve food will have at least one salad on the menu and if not then the chef will more than likely be happy to make one for you. When you do order salad, remember to request the dressing on the side to avoid having your meal delivered with an unhealthy amount already drizzled on top.

If you don't always want to eat salad then look through the menu to find simple dishes that are made from fresh or raw ingredients. Even if a restaurant doesn't seem to offer too many healthy options, they will usually have a selection of vegetable side dishes that you can combine to create a healthy and filling main meal.

Another thing to look out for is dishes that are freshly made because that way they are less likely to be full of harmful preservatives. These might range from plastic contaminants to other chemicals, or even excessive amounts of sodium. I generally advise that it is best to avoid packaged foods where possible and dining out is no exception. If the menu doesn't specify whether the dish has been made fresh then your waiter or waitress will be able to let you know. It is also a common practice in restaurants to use salt, butter, and refined oils to improve the flavor of a recipe. Again, you can always ask the person serving you how the dish has been prepared to avoid this.

> When eating out, watch out for any menu items described as "crispy," "scalloped," "Alfredo," "gratin," and "pan fried"—all indicators of an unhealthy choice!

Rule 2: Grilled or steamed, but not fried

Checking to see how a dish has been cooked will be of endless help to your diet efforts. Eating a plate of vegetables will be of detriment to any diet, if they have been fried in refined oils. The food in question will absorb fat from the oil and that can make a healthy option end up with a high fat content. When we consume high levels of unhealthy fat our blood cholesterol levels increase and our arteries can become clogged over time. As the blood flow becomes restricted, we are then at a higher risk of high blood pressure, strokes, type 2 diabetes, and heart disease. Opt instead for grilled or steamed dishes because these will be much lower in fat than their fried counterparts.

When foods are fried they usually cook at a much higher temperature than when grilled and steamed. Nutrients are easily destroyed when exposed to high temperatures and will rapidly lose their health benefits. However, when you grill a food, the excess fat usually drips away meaning more vitamins and minerals will be retained. Grilling will also help to seal in moisture, which helps to flavor the food, making it less likely that, any additional butter, salt, or oil will be deemed necessary.

Steaming is another great option when it comes to cooking and is one of the healthiest ways to do so. Nutrient loss is minimal and the structure and the flavor of the food in less effected. Although some people think steaming is generally only used to prepare vegetables, you can in fact cook almost anything in a steamer. Additionally, no oil is required for steaming, which means your meal will be much lower in calories than if you were to fry it.

It may not always be noted on the menu how a dish has been prepared so it is always worth checking before you order.

Rule 3: Nix the starch (a.k.a. the bread basket), dressings, and sauces

Even in a healthy restaurant you can soon consume a large amount of calories when you indulge in the added extras. The three biggest culprits when it comes to this are the bread basket on your table, as well as the dressings and sauce that you add to your meal.

Avoiding the bread basket might be easier said than done but it is not impossible! If you know that you are going to be waiting a while for your meal then make sure you have a small piece of fruit or a handful of nuts before you go. Not only will this help you to steer clear of the bread but research has also shown that eating an apple before a meal can aid in weight loss.[1,2] It is thought that the pectin found in apples will prevent the body from absorbing as much fat as it usually would. Pectin is also known to be an appetite suppressant, which will mean you are likely to eat less during your meal and if you're not starving hungry then you'll find it much easier to wait for your meal without diving into the bread basket!

If you order a salad and then cover it in dressing, this is the same concept as eating that plate of vegetables that has been fried in refined oils. You are essentially taking a healthy dish and making it incredibly bad for your health. The majority of dressings are high in fat and calories, and you should never be adding more than one or two tablespoons at a maximum.

Sauces like tomato ketchup, mayonnaise, and BBQ sauce might immediately come to mind when you think of eating certain meals. Maybe you can't even imagine eating your favorite dish without adding a large dollop of mayonnaise or ketchup first, but doing so can add up to a lot of extra calories and added sugar, too! Even though you might argue that you are enhancing the flavor of your meal and thereby increasing how much you are going to enjoy it, the truth is that you are probably just doing so out of habit. Best to enjoy these sauces at home with a wholesome, homemade ketchup, BBQ sauce, and mayonnaise so that you know exactly what's going into them.

Rule 4: Drink water before your meal

Keeping hydrated is great for weight loss, the appearance of your skin, the health of your cells, and your energy levels among many other things. Regularly drinking water through the day is important but drinking a glass of water immediately before a meal can be beneficial to health.

Weight loss is one of the most sought after benefits of drinking water before a meal. Drinking water can create a sense of fullness, which means you'll tend to consume fewer calories, but it will also hydrate you so you're less likely to choose a calorie-loaded beverage to go with your food.

Stress and genetics both play a part in the appearance of your skin but adequate hydration is also a huge contributing factor. Make it a habit to drink a glass of water before each meal and you be improving the health of your skin effortlessly.

We have up to a trillion cells in our bodies and taking care of them is essential for optimum health. In order for our cells to stay healthy, nutrients have to be able to get in while toxins must be able to be removed effectively. This process of nutrients entering and toxins leaving is known as "cell turnover," and plays a huge part in good health. As well as providing nourishment itself, water also carries nutrients into cells, making it doubly important to drink up!

Water is one of the main sources of energy for the body and it is always a better idea to be constantly hydrated instead of waiting until you get thirsty. By waiting until you are thirsty you are allowing your energy stores to become depleted and this will also often mean you don't drink enough water throughout the day. Not drinking enough water means you'll urinate less and this can be a bad thing for your kidneys. The process of urination removes certain toxins from the body that have been filtered by the kidneys.

If your urine is colorless then it's a good sign that you're drinking enough water, however, if it's yellow or darker then you need more hydration.

Rule 5: The one-for-one rule

When you go out for a meal it is much easier to give into the temptation of an alcoholic drink than if you were at home. Good company, a great atmosphere, and the feeling of being out treating yourself can make it easy to get carried away with alcohol. If you want to enjoy yourself without too many restrictions then the best thing to do is to get strategic with your drinks. Stick to the "one-for-one rule," which basically means you drink a glass of water after every alcoholic beverage you have. Make sure that you don't order another alcoholic drink until you have finished the glass of water—no cheating! The additional water will help your body to metabolize the alcohol and to keep you hydrated during the night.

One of healthiest drinks you can choose from the drinks menu is red wine. It is rich in antioxidants and promotes cardiovascular health[3,4] because of the wealth of resveratrol contained within. On the other side of the spectrum are cocktails, such as margaritas and pina coladas, both of which are laden with calories. You might not find it at every establishment but sake is one of my favorites when it comes to making healthy alcohol choices. Sake is a Japanese dry wine made from fermented rice and is believed to contribute to cardiovascular health. It is slightly higher in alcohol percentage than most wines and can be enjoyed hot, chilled, or at room temperature.

Take these five Simple Rules when eating out and then use your Flexi-Five when you're not, and you'll be well on your way to healthy eating for life.

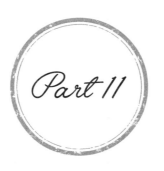

Part 11

Simple Rules
for Happiness
and Unstoppable
Energy

*W*hat if, instead of thinking about solving your whole life, you just think about adding additional good things—one at a time? Just let your pile of good things grow.

Chapter 8

Channel Your Superhero Powers

Learn how and why to include meditation, breathing, affirmations, and yoga easily and effortlessly in your life every day.

I can't stress enough how important these four activities are in my life. They have become like my four children—the other four superhero powers in my life. I can honestly say, hand on heart, that without them I would not be the person I am today. Making a conscious effort to implement them into my daily life was at first tough—I will be completely honest here—because I thought I was too busy. Well, and truth be told, I am super busy, which is even more reason to put them into practice as much as I can. I finally realized that putting these activities into my daily routine helped me profoundly, especially during those crazy, hectic, and incredibly stressful days. My only question to myself right now is: "What took me so long?"

The more we get crazy busy, the more stress we have, and the less happy we are. But do you know what stress can do to your body and mind? I didn't until I started really researching it and really truly understanding how these superhero powers can keep that stress away!

Some not-so-very side effects of stress on you!

When you let it get the better of you, stress can seem to infiltrate every part of your life. It can have several negative health effects that can soon add up to a much bigger problem.

Frequent headaches are a common symptom of stress and masking this symptom with painkillers won't really do you any good because as soon as the medication subsides, the problem still exists. Hair loss is another common, but quite scary side effect of stress. As well as falling out in specific areas, your hair can also become generally thinner as a result of high stress. This is of course something most of us would want to avoid. Acne can also appear during periods of high stress, which can then cause people to worry about their appearance, leading to more stress! But as with anything, if you get these symptoms, it's worth paying a visit to your medical practitioner for a check up.

It may surprise you to know that your memory function can also be negatively affected by stress. This is due to damage caused to the glutamate receptors. Insomnia is also a common problem among the highly stressed and will lead to a whole fresh set of health complaints, if it persists. It may sound dramatic but heart attacks are much more common among those who live in stress mode.

As well as affecting your general health in less than favorable ways, stress also quickly leads to weight gain for a number of reasons. First, it can cause cravings for sugary, fatty, comfort foods. These foods usually have no nutritional value and don't really provide any comfort or relief from the stress; however, we still continue to turn to them! Studies have also found that elevated amounts of the stress hormone cortisol is linked to excess fat in the abdomen region, meaning if you are stressed out then it is likely that you will find it harder to shift that belly fat.[1,2]

> Elevated cortisol levels are also linked to chronic back pain, which can really impact your quality of life.

Finally, your immune system and the function of your adrenal glands can both be impaired by stress. This means that you are much more likely to get ill and experience fatigue.

With so many health concerns being posed by stress, it is amazing to me that more people are not making every attempt to eradicate it from their lives! Stress is, of course, a natural reaction to a difficult or challenging situation and the production of stress hormones occurs to help us deal with the situation.

However, as our lives have become increasingly busy and hectic, we are being put in more and more of these stressful situations, leading to excessive amounts of adrenalin and cortisol coursing through our bodies. Many thousands of years ago these stressful situations were more likely to be due to coming across a wild animal that might want to eat us, as opposed to the modern-day stresses of finances and job expectations. The stress hormones were intended to help give us the strength and the stamina to get out of dangerous situations unscathed. Although this is not applicable in the modern world in the same way, the reaction in our body is still the same.

Sit back and take stock of that stress

As well as the stress that occurs in everyday life, we are also inflicting it upon ourselves in other ways. When we overeat, oversleep, behave irresponsibly, smoke, drink, or argue with loved ones, we are inevitably giving ourselves a huge bundle of stress to deal with—whether we realize it or not!

You might not even realize how stressed out you are until you sit back and take stock of your life. If you notice that you complain a lot, never seem to have any free time, or if you feel unhappy a lot of the time (in work, relationships, or family life) believing that eventually the suffering will bring a positive result, then the chances are you have let stress take over your life.

First of all, everybody loves to complain sometimes and venting your frustration is in fact good for you! But if you are always complaining then something has to give! Address the issues that are upsetting you and find constructive resolutions.

Second, people who are stressed out often go through life on autopilot. They move from one task to the next, believing that they have to be busy in order to feel productive and fulfilled. Take a time out and find some space for yourself. Relaxation is key to a well-balanced life, and once you stop trying to force yourself to enjoy activities and pursuits that you really have no interest in, your stress levels will lower.

Finally, suffering through unhappiness does nobody any good. If you are unhappy in your relationship, chances are your partner is, too. If you are having trouble adjusting at work, or if there is tension at home, then simply talking the issue out with the relevant people can often make a huge difference.

> Never settle for unhappiness because then you devalue yourself and tell the world that this is all you want from life—what could be more stressful than that?

So, make time to combat stress by incorporating these superhero powers into your daily life.

Meditation

Meditating for even just a couple of minutes each day can truly help to bring a sense of focus into your life. It can be difficult to find the motivation and the time to meditate at first, but once you get into the routine you'll be happy that you overcame the initial hurdles!

> "Go within every day and find the inner strength so that the world will not blow your candle out."
> KATHERINE DUNHAM

Meditation embodies a range of practices that all serve to encourage relaxation as well as the growth of patience, compassion, forgiveness, and gratitude. At its core, meditation is a practice that provides rest to the mind and creates a distance from the stresses and worries of everyday life. It enables a different sense of consciousness to that which is usually experienced and will promote an enhanced sense of calm wellbeing.

Make a commitment to spend just a few minutes meditating at first and then work to increase this time. It is important that you try to fulfill your commitment to meditate every day—again even if it's just a FEW minutes—but if you miss a day then you can soon get yourself back on track.

Finding a peaceful, comfortable place to meditate will help you to enjoy this process. However, it is, of course, possible to meditate absolutely anywhere. If you know that your evening will be chaotic once you arrive home from work then a couple of private moments of meditation on your office floor could be a great place to start. Eventually finding a permanent space that you can associate with your meditation will really help you to become more connected to the practice. For me, I either meditate first thing in the morning before my kids wake up for school or grab a juice, find a spot, and sit still for few minutes with my eyes closed. That's how simple it can be!

Barriers to meditation

A common barrier to meditation is a hectic family life. Inviting your children or partner to practice with you is the perfect solution to this. You may find that your family begins to enjoy it and will continue to do so with you. If they decide that meditation is not for them, then at least having experienced it will show them why you need to take this time for yourself and encourage them to give you the time and space to do so.

It is completely normal for your mind to wander at first and counting slowly down from 10 is a good way to get started. Every time you're distracted by a thought begin this counting again to get yourself back on track. It also helps to pay close attention to your breathing, as this leaves no space for other thoughts.

> Breathe gently in and out through your nose and hear the silence all around you.

It is important to avoid seeing meditation as something else that you have to do during the day. If it starts to feel like a chore then re-evaluate why you are doing it in the first place. You have to remember that it is an action that contributes to your general wellbeing, not something to feel negative about!

Bringing meditation into every day

Getting into a regular practice of meditation will enable you to feel its full benefits of and there are a few things you can do to make sure you stick to it.

First of all, picking a set time during your day to meditate will allow it to become a solid part of your routine. If you know that your days are usually chaotic once you step out of the front door, then meditating in the early morning is probably the best time for you. That way you approach the day having already equipped yourself with the peace and focus you need. This also means that you are less likely to decide not to do it after a long day, if you had it scheduled in for the evening.

If, like many people, you are already on a tight schedule, then set a gentle alarm so that you meditate for a pre-determined amount of time. Even just three minutes is fine if that is all you can manage! By setting an alarm you won't have to worry that you are spending too much time meditating, if you know you have things you need to attend to. This then leaves your mind free to pay full attention to the task at hand—relaxation and mindfulness!

Second, having a persistent focal point on which to center your meditation will encourage you to develop a sense of consistency. To start with it is a good choice to focus on your breathing, as this requires some concentration. As your practice develops, you might also try focusing on the sounds that come to you as you meditate. It is also helpful to have your goals and ambitions in your mind, whether they are short- or long-term ones. If you find your mind starts to drift away from these specific thoughts then pull yourself back to the present moment and start again.

Finally, having realistic expectations of yourself and your practice is key to staying on track. If you put too much pressure on the process then you are inevitably going to end up feeling disappointed. It is not reasonable to expect to feel the benefits of meditation after just a few sessions. Over time, as your practice continues and your attitude toward it develops, you will naturally experience a shift in the way you approach your days, and the way in which you engage with the world. Even if you feel as though you don't feel a difference in your frame of mind when you are meditating, you will soon notice how better equipped you are away from the floor.

When you need to bring some peace and relaxation into your day, meditation can be a very effective tool. With just a few short minutes of practice you can work toward restoring the natural balance in your body and promote a greater sense of calm.

Learning to meditate

In the exercises that follow you'll see how important breathing is to achieving an effective meditation practice. It is absolutely normal for your mind to drift to other thoughts when you are meditating and being able to re-focus yourself depends on being able to bring your attention back to your breath. That said, it is important not to give yourself a hard time when this happens and, instead, take another deep breath and concentrate on the flow of air coming in and out of your body.

Simple meditation *Exercise*

Find a place to sit, where you can relax and won't be disturbed. You can spend as little or as much time as you choose, but about three minutes is about right when starting out. So once you are comfortable, set an alarm for three minutes then close your eyes and just continue to breathe normally for a few moments. On the next breath, try to feel your breath coming into your belly and focus on this thought for three breaths, in and out. After these three breaths, move your breathing focus up into your chest and breathe this way for three breaths, in and out. Repeat this sequence of breathing first in your belly and then in your chest until your alarm goes off to tell you to stop. That's how simple it is! And I think you'll find that these three minutes out of your day are extremely effective, too!

Breathing

Breathing exercises are an incredibly powerful tool for relaxation and promoting mindfulness. Consciously addressing your breathing will help you to become more present and aware of your surroundings.

She had a revolutionary idea: She would make more time for life's truly important things. First on the list: Breathing

Focusing on your breathing forces you to pay absolute attention to what you are doing in that moment, and that is essential for entering the right frame of mind for meditation. If you find that you struggle to keep your mind clear while you are meditating then finding a breathing exercise that works for you is a great solution.

The following exercise is simple but effective. It teaches you how to breathe from your diaphragm and that encourages the abdominal muscles to expand. When the muscles expand in this way they contract around your organs, which improves the digestive process.

Abdominal breathing *Exercise*

To begin, sit up straight, either in a chair or on the floor, and place your hands on your stomach. Then inhale through your nose and follow that breath with your mind into your stomach, which should expand outward. As you exhale, again through your nose, bring your stomach inward and upward. Try mentally counting to four on the inhalation, pressing the belly into the hand and exhaling for four, pressing the belly back toward the spine.

Repeat this breathing pattern for a few minutes at first and then extend the amount of time as your practice develops.

I use this abdominal breathing technique before a big meeting, when I'm stressed, stuck in traffic, on the school run, when I have too many to-dos, I am in the midst of drama or crisis, and even before I go to bed!

Once you have mastered abdominal breathing, give the following exercise a try. It is slightly more advanced and is the next step in your breathing practice. This three-part breathing exercise is commonly used during yoga practice. It utilizes the chest as well as your stomach and ribs. The intention of this exercise is to encourage optimum oxygen flow through the body to bring about feelings of calm.

Mindful breathing *Exercise*

To start this exercise, sit in a comfortable position on the floor with your spine straight. Your eyes should be closed and your face should be as relaxed as possible. As you breathe in, soften your stomach and ribs and push them out slightly. As you come to the end of this inhalation, feel your chest rise also. Hold your breath for a few counts and then, as you exhale, push your chest back down and bring your stomach and ribs back inward. Continue breathing in this way for four or five minutes, always with your stomach extending, ribs expanding and chest rising on the inhale, and the opposite on the exhale.

The duo effort of focusing on your breath, as well as the actions of your body, can help to really channel your concentration. This is particularly useful for combatting anxiety, depression, and insomnia—especially if practiced for longer periods of time. It is difficult for your mind to wander as you do this breathing exercise, and that can help you to regain a sense of mental clarity—which is essential in keeping negative thoughts and destructive behaviors from our minds. You will be teaching your brain to deal with the stresses in life in a productive and sensible way while also aligning yourself internally.

> Mindful breathing requires you to be completely present in the here and now, and is a great way to harness your focus.

Using your breath to find more calm and positivity

Focusing just on your breath is incredibly useful if you find yourself struggling to pay attention or if negative thoughts are infiltrating your mind. As you begin a breathing exercise, your mind is forced to concentrate on the breaths you take and the pace at which they come in and out of your nose or mouth. This leaves little room for anything else—negativity included!

Even though our breathing takes care of itself with little attention from us during most of the day, we can sometimes experience shallow breathing without realizing it. This is usually due to stress and is a big warning sign that you need to bring some relaxation into your life. Shallow breathing can stimulate a certain part of the nervous system that then signals to the body to produce more stress hormones. This is obviously the exact opposite of what we want.

Breathing mindfully and deeply stimulates the nervous system to promote a state of relaxation throughout the mind and body.

Knowing when to turn to mindful breathing can really help you to avoid making certain situations much worse. For example, if you are having an argument with a colleague or loved one then taking a moment to focus on your breathing, instead of continuing to engage in the argument, can help to clear your mind and prevent you from saying something you don't mean. Even just a few deep breaths in and out can give you the time to readjust your attitude and proceed with calm and logic.

Affirmations

When you need a dose of inspiration or motivation, focusing on one or more affirmations can really help to get you on track. Affirmations can be a powerful tool to aid spiritual, emotional, and physical development but when using them try to really make the effort to completely connect with them. In doing so, you will work toward eliminating negative thought patterns and this can really help to change certain unconscious behaviors (including bad eating habits, such as sugar addiction).

If you have issues with loving and caring for yourself then using affirmations can help you to embrace the mindfulness necessary to work past this and embrace self-love. Affirmations are also great for learning how to appropriately deal with and manage stress, especially when used in conjunction with meditation.

At a very basic level, an affirmation is a statement that enables positivity, motivation, and inspiration. You can either say this statement out loud, in your mind, or even write it down. I would recommend that you choose to say them out loud when you feel comfortable doing so, as this allows it to have a bigger impact on the mind. It also makes it much easier for you to commit to memory so that it leaves an imprint in your mind during the rest of your day.

> Your chosen affirmations must be applicable to you and your experience. It is pointless focusing on things that are not relevant to your life or out of your control.

When choosing an affirmation to focus on, try to choose something that isn't too long. A short sentence that you can easily say over and over again will help to keep your attention on it. I also suggest that you make using the affirmation your prime task. Make sure you are free of distractions, such as in a peaceful, meditative state, or during an exercise or even a work break. Bring your mind into the present moment and be mindful of your breathing. Once you have said your affirmation once, allow yourself a few seconds to let it sink in before you repeat it.

You don't have to say the same affirmation every day and it is useful to have a list that you call upon during your week for some variation. If you have one or two things that you particularly want to work on, such as weight loss or stress, then it is best to constantly choose affirmations that are connected to these things.

Bringing more of what you want toward you

When you use affirmations regularly you are essentially re-programming your brain to strive for the things that you want. It brings your goals and desires to the forefront of your mind and you will start to pay much more attention to these things in your day to day. So if you use an affirmation that promotes self-worth and self-love then you are going to notice positive things about yourself that you might usually overlook.

Using affirmations that suggest that your goals have already been attained is an even more powerful way to use this positive thinking tool. For example, if you use the affirmation, "I am happy and content with every aspect of my life," but there are certain areas that you feel could use an improvement, then you will be more motivated to work toward making your affirmation a reality. The same is also true of body image. For example if you use the affirmation, "I love my body how it is and I am my ideal weight," but in fact you know you still have a couple of pounds to lose to reach your goal, then you'll find that you have more drive to do so.

> Ask for what you want and be prepared to get it!
>
> Maya Angelou

There is a certain amount of debate as to how long it takes for a chosen affirmation to really make a dent in your mind. Generally speaking you should start to notice a difference in your attitude after a few weeks of daily affirmations that will continue to shift as time goes on.

Affirmations to get you going *Exercise*

Here are some examples that you can use or tailor to make them more specific to your experience:

* *I let go of people who do not have my best interests at heart.*
* *I love my body and appreciate all that it does for me.*
* *Every day I grow as a person and learn new things.*
* *The longest relationship I have in my life is with me.*

* *I have confidence in my own ability to be the best I can be.*
* *I am a gift to the world and I will not waste time on self-pity and sadness.*
* *I forgive my own mistakes and those of the people I love.*
* *Any hardships I have endured have made me a stronger and better person.*
* *Worries are a drain on my energy and I choose to let them go instead.*
* *This day will bring me nothing but joy and happiness.*

As you say each affirmation, try to visualize yourself and your life once you have reached the goal you have in mind.

Yoga

For me, yoga is a fully integral part of my life. It's one of those things that I now believe I really can't live without. It's definitely made me a better person, friend, mother, and wife, and is something that I will do for the rest of my life because of the enormous physical, mental, and emotional benefits it brings me. Of course, it's well documented that yoga helps lower stress and improve flexibility, and these are both great reasons to practice yoga. However, there are many more health benefits to yoga that you might not be aware of.

First of all, studies have shown that yoga can have an influence over our cravings for food.[3,4] It is believed that yoga promotes a stronger mind-body connection, which better equips us to understand what our body needs. In real terms this means when we experience unhealthy cravings, we are more likely to make positive food choices.

Second, your digestive system can benefit massively from regular yoga practice. Several of the poses serve as a kind of internal massage for your digestive system and associated organs, helping to alleviate any bloating, indigestion, or constipation you might be experiencing. Your immune system will also soon feel the effects of yoga as the breathing techniques increase blood flow to your organs, which helps to provide them with ample oxygen.

If you experience pain in a particular area of your body, then a trained yogi can help you to tailor your yoga practice to address this complaint. Once you pinpoint the specific problem you can use a series of poses, twists, and holds to target the affected area. Yoga can help you to regain full function while also improving flexibility and strength. This will then help to prevent the complaint from returning.

> Yoga enables us to become more in tune with the body so we notice pains and irregularities with greater ease.

The great thing about yoga is that there is always a class to suit your specific level. You don't need to stress about not being fit enough or not being able to keep up, as your practice is unique to you. It is an inclusive form of exercise that promotes acceptance of your true self. It teaches you to work toward progress instead of perfection. You will notice the small wins, as you're able to hold poses for longer and take your stretches further.

Tuning in to your body

As time progresses your understanding of your own body will develop, too. You will come to realize that your body is only as strong as every individual part of you and that you need your body to work in sync with your mind to progress. This is a concept that you will then begin to apply to other areas of your life, encouraging you to work on the small parts of the whole in order to create a happier you.

At first yoga might seem to be just another exercise, a go-to activity to get fit. But after a few sessions you'll begin to understand the spiritual nature of this practice and how it teaches us to find a deeper connection with ourselves.

The combination of meditation and breathing in yoga can truly help you to learn self-discipline and a greater understanding of your own presence. As your body gets used to this new addition to your routine, you might discover that it is more physically challenging than you envisioned. Far from being a reason to quit before you have really even started, you should embrace this new challenge and overcome each and every obstacle as you come to it. I like to think of it as "goal setting" and that's a good thing for you, your body, your mind, and your spirit.

There is SO much to be discovered while practicing yoga and a great deal to benefit from. While we are on the mat, the strength, flexibility and stamina of our bodies is increasing and our patience and mindfulness is growing. However, the lessons of yoga don't stop when we leave the studio and the things we learn on the mat extend into several other corners of our lives.

As our bodies adjust to a yoga practice we will often feel the aches and pains that naturally occur as muscles stretch and grow. The result of this is that we become stronger and better equipped to make it through the next lesson. This also teaches us to accept the challenges in life that we must overcome. Often these challenges can seem too difficult or distressing to work past but when you do manage to move forward, the experience makes you a stronger person.

> Yoga is a personal evolution that equips us to deal with future burdens, stresses, and dramas.

Even after a relatively short amount of practice you'll find that your body becomes more flexible and with it your attitude and mental stamina because yoga teaches us that we are resilient and able to adjust when life takes an unexpected turn. As our bodies can be flexible, so too can be our approach to confrontation and adversity.

Finally, the breathing techniques that we learn in a yoga session also show us the importance of expelling negativity from our lives. As we breathe in we are summoning clearing, cleansing, and even healing energy and focus into our bodies and minds, and as we exhale we release the stresses and negativities that we collect throughout the day. Knowing when to breathe out is the same as knowing when to let go of the things that cause us distress.

Essential yoga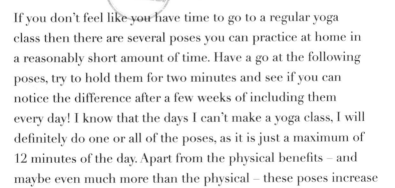

If you don't feel like you have time to go to a regular yoga class then there are several poses you can practice at home in a reasonably short amount of time. Have a go at the following poses, try to hold them for two minutes and see if you can notice the difference after a few weeks of including them every day! I know that the days I can't make a yoga class, I will definitely do one or all of the poses, as it is just a maximum of 12 minutes of the day. Apart from the physical benefits – and maybe even much more than the physical – these poses increase my mood, make me happy, calm me down, but at the same time they energize me, too.

Downward Facing Dog (*Adho Mukha Svanasana*)

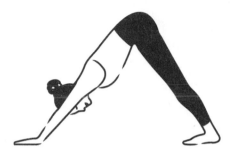

The most comfortable way to get into this pose is to begin on the floor on your hands and knees. Then push your tailbone up into the air as you tuck your toes under. Try to shift your weight on to your heels as you come into the pose. Your body will form a triangle-like shape as you let your head naturally point down toward the floor.

This pose is great for stretching out your back and you can make the bend more intense by tucking your chin up toward your chest and bending your knees slightly. This will cause your chest and shoulders to open, which is a great relief if you have been sitting still for a long time during the day.

Through natural everyday actions, our calves and hamstrings can become quite tight. The muscles in the back can also get stiff and tense during the day and this pose is perfect to unwind all three. As you continue your practice it will also increase the strength of your ankles and wrists. Striving to improve strength in these joints is essential as we age if we want to prevent injury and weakness.

If you can feel tension in your neck and shoulders then gently shaking your head from side to side while you hold this pose can really help. When you have held the pose for several breaths you can return to your hands and knees to comfortably get out of the pose.

Standing Forward Bend (*Uttanasana*)

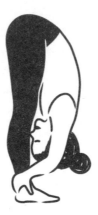

To do this pose you simply need to stand with your legs hip-width apart and bend over from the hip. Bring your torso forward without arching your back and reach toward the floor. Hold this pose for five breaths before returning to a standing position, and repeat as you like.

This pose has many of the same benefits as *Viparita Karani*, described later (*see page 190*), such the increase in blood flow and the release of the lower back muscles. This pose also helps to engage your hip muscles and by using them you are encouraging them to regenerate with fresh bone cells and cartilage.

Doing this pose puts the body into a position that you don't usually naturally do so it is a great way to remind dormant muscles that they still have work to do! As the body extends into the pose, pressure will be relieved from your spine and you will eventually be able to lengthen the back with complete comfort.

Squat Pose (*Malasana*)

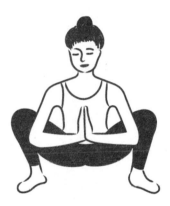

To do this pose you simply lower your body into the squatting position and hold the pose. You can also bring your hands together in front of your body in prayer position.

The hip joints benefit most from the squat pose as it can help to retain and improve flexibility. As we get older the movement we have in the hips can quickly diminish so it is important that we work to preserve it. Unfortunately, modern-day jobs call for us to spend more and more time sitting still and leaning toward our desks or steering wheels. This causes the muscles in our legs, backs, shoulders, and necks to tighten and they become restricted over time. The alignment of the rest of your body also relies on your hips, most noticeably when you are standing still or walking.

As well as relieving muscle tension and strengthening the hips, the squat pose is also beneficial to our internal organs. As you move into and hold the pose, you will be stimulating your organs, which helps to reinforce their function. Regular movement also helps them to retain their elasticity and promotes a healthy circulatory system.

Mountain Pose (*Tadasana*)

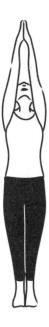

By standing tall with your feet together and shoulders relaxed you can easily enter the mountain pose. Hold your arms at your side and, as you breathe in, raise them straight above your head with your palms facing together.

This pose is perfect for correcting your posture as well as improving stability. It can also be particularly beneficial if you have a recent injury to the shoulders or any tension in that area. This is because as you move into the pose and hold it, you are letting go of this tension and encouraging relaxation and flexibility instead.

Triangle Pose (*Trikonasana*)

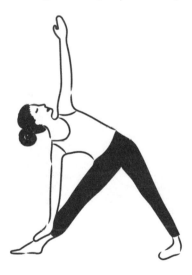

Stand with your feet slightly further apart than your hips and move your right toes to face out while the left toes face inward at a 90-degree angle. Keep both of your legs straight and bend at the hip toward your right leg. Continue moving your torso as far to the right as you can and then place your right hand just above your ankle as you extend the left arm over your shoulder. Take 10 breaths while you hold this pose and then spin your right hip forward and left hip back as you hold for 10 more breaths.

This pose is perfect for strengthening and stretching the ankles, knees, hips, calves, shoulders and thighs. It also stimulates the organs in the abdomen, relieving stress and improving digestion.

Legs-up-the-Wall Pose (*Viparita Karani*)

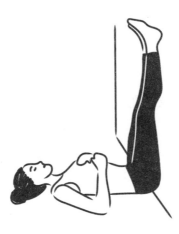

All you need to do to accomplish this pose is to lie on your back with your legs positioned up the wall in front of you. The easiest way to get into the pose is to sit with your right side against the wall and then gently swing your legs up as your head and shoulders come down gently to rest on the floor. As you hold this pose, place one hand on your abdomen and the other over your chest. Then, as you breathe deeply in and out, be aware of the natural rhythm of your breathing and body.

This is a restorative pose that is great for relaxation. In fact, if you practice it regularly before bed then it can help to improve the quality and duration of your sleep. It is not intended as an intense stretch for the legs so if you feel your hamstrings pulling then move into a more comfortable position. Many people find it quite helpful to place a rolled up towel or cushion under their neck.

This pose is useful for reducing inflammation in your feet and ankles. Once you have held this pose for a few moments, you will also notice that you feel a light stretch in your hamstring, which helps to relax the lower back muscles. Over time this pose aids blood flow to the digestive system, heart, lungs, and brain.

When you use meditation, breathing, yoga, and affirmations all together in your everyday life, even if for just a couple of minutes each day, you will soon notice an increased sense of calm and relaxation, self-confidence, and self-love. And not only will your body move with greater ease but your mind will be better equipped to deal with the stresses and problems that life throws at you. And for me, it's all about being the best version of myself. I mean, let's face it, there is only one of you... there will be never be another you, so might as well be the best you can be.

Chapter 9

Easy Tips to Keep You Going...

Learn what, how, and why to include vitamin D, water, greens, movement, mindfulness, and sleep to get that unstoppable energy.

Give me more energy! That is what we have been trying to do for as long as humans have been around! Way back in the day, we would get our energy from whole foods, including chia seeds (yes, they have been around since 3,500BCE.) But fast forward to the present day and we are overexposed to a plethora of energy drinks, waters, and powders containing unnatural ingredients, which cause a very low "low" after the initial "high".

The need for energy is exploding because of our increasingly busy and hectic lives, but luckily so is the health and wellness industry, which hypes up the education of finding energy the wholesome way. I get asked nearly every single day... how do you do it all with four kids, teaching yoga, cycling everywhere, writing, blogging, and so on and so on. And where do you find the energy? So here are my top tips to stay "high" on life in the most perfect way.

Get your vitamin D

Making sure you get out in the sunshine is a good way to naturally keep your energy levels up. Natural sunlight also reduces levels of stress hormones in the body and lowers your blood pressure. Additionally, getting an adequate amount of sun will encourage serotonin production, which means great things for your energy and for your mood. Many people, especially office workers, begin to get drowsy in the afternoon. A brisk walk out in the sun for just a few minutes can help you to overcome this and get your focus back.

The optimum health of your bones and teeth also relies on getting an adequate amount of vitamin D. Although calcium is the main element of bone and teeth health, calcium can only be properly absorbed when there is a sufficient amount of certain nutrients present in the body. Vitamin D is one of these nutrients and it increases the amount of calcium the body can use. As this process helps to nourish and strengthen your bones it will also enable growth. Having strong and healthy bones will help to protect you against injury and age-related degeneration that can lead to problems such as osteoporosis.

Your immune system has a lot to gain from a healthy dose of vitamin D—it helps with maintenance and regulation of the immune system cells, as well as the nervous system.

Although endless amounts of sunshine sounds like a great thing, vitamin D is a fat-soluble vitamin. This means that if you are exposed to too much sun, or consume an excessive amount in your diet, then it can have harmful effects. However, this is not a common problem, whereas deficiencies of vitamin D are becoming more widespread due to the use of sunscreens. If you regularly spend time outside and eat a well-balanced and varied diet abundant in plant-based options, then you will usually have no need to take this vitamin as a supplement unless pregnant or breastfeeding.

Take a water break

Dehydration is one of the most common causes of fatigue. Making sure you take regular water breaks throughout your day can help to keep you functioning well. Water aids energy production within our cells as well as many other important functions. Additionally, not only does it provide an effective energy boost when you drink it, but when splashed on your face it can also stimulate your circulation, which will help to wake you up.

The concept of hydration can be understood in simple terms as the process in the body by which water is managed, both in relation to metabolic function and perspiration. The presence of water in the body enables nutrients to be carried around the body to the cells that need them. It also means that toxins are able to leave the body through sweating and urination.

When there is not an adequate amount of water present in the body we can quickly become sleepy and disorientated, it is also common to feel hungry and suffer from headaches and low blood pressure.

It is generally suggested that we need eight glasses of water every day. However, if you feel like you need more than this, then absolutely drink more.

Literally every cell in the body contains water and your body is approximately 70 percent water—essential for us to function properly yet often overlooked. Always carry a bottle with you and you will never be caught short.

Drink something green

Taking a break from your day to get a healthy green drink into your body is often a great way to quickly feel refreshed. Making your own juice with a juicer or a smoothie in the blender is the best way to get a huge dose of nutrient goodness into your system.

Kale, spinach, and kiwis are particularly perfect when it comes to making healthy, green drinks.

I like to focus on green fruits and vegetables in particular because they get their fantastic color from chlorophyll. During the process of photosynthesis these plants utilize the energy of the sun and we have a lot to gain from including these plants in our diet.

If you don't always eat a varied diet full of wholesome goodness then you might be deficient in certain nutrients. Juices and smoothies, especially the ones you make yourself, can contain several different health-boosting ingredients. This means that you are getting a massive dose of nutrition in a relatively small serving.

Choosing to have a smoothie first thing in the morning is one of the best breakfast choices you can make! You can easily customize your smoothie every day so that you always have something new and interesting to look forward to. It is perfect for those of us who are super busy and need to eat on the go but also great to sit down with and enjoy slowly as you prepare for the day ahead. The huge dose of nutrients that you give yourself with every smoothie means you will always go into your day with the energy that your body needs!

Natural green teas are also a good option and are favored for their high antioxidant count. When you drink green tea regularly you are not only giving your energy levels a boost, but also your metabolic function and your immune system. If you drink coffee throughout the day to make yourself more alert then substituting a green drink for your coffee is a great idea. This swap will give you a kick-start without the inevitable crash that comes with caffeine.

Move and stretch

Sitting down for extended periods of time is one of the unhealthiest things that we do in our modern age. Studies have revealed that the average person sits down for almost eight hours every day.[1,2] After sitting for just one hour, the production of fat-burning enzymes declines by up to 90 percent. When you do this, your metabolism is also negatively affected, which then has a knock-on effect on levels of HDL cholesterol in the body.

Extended periods of sitting down have been linked to heart disease, diabetes, cancer, and of course obesity.[3,4]

If you have a job that requires you to sit down to work then make sure you are taking regular breaks to walk around and stretch for a few minutes. Setting an alarm to go off on the hour, every hour, is a great prompt to do so. As you move around you will encourage the natural flow of energy and endorphins around your body, improving both your energy and your mood.

Stay present

Feeling as though you are going through your day on autopilot is certainly not a unique feeling. So many of us have repetitive routines that can rapidly curb our motivation, causing boredom to set in. When this happens we are prone to distractions and feelings of disconnection. To keep our energy levels up it is important that we approach our days in a mindful way and remind ourselves of the reasons why we do the things we do. It is by no means a bad thing to think about the past and contemplate the future but when you have a task to complete, whether that is at work or at home, then staying present will help to keep you focused and on track why you do it.

> Try to stay present during your day, instead of letting your mind wander to stressful thoughts.

As we explored in detail in the previous chapter, extended periods of stress can be incredibly detrimental to our wellbeing and quickly lead to fatigue and illness. If you have worries or concerns then you need to set aside time to deal with and resolve them.

> There is nothing to be gained from dwelling on stressful thoughts and a lot of energy and positivity to lose!

High levels of stress will certainly sap your energy levels and avoiding negative situations and toxic relationships is key to combatting this. If you are someone who is guilty of shutting their emotions out, as opposed to dealing with them then you will more than likely find that these emotions creep up on you during your day to day. When this happens you can become overwhelmed with having to get through your day as well as tackle these uninvited thoughts.

Practicing mindfulness is a great way to overcome this and to bring your full attention back to where it needs to be. You need to inspire yourself to pay attention to what is happening in the present and drive yourself to commit to what you are doing 100 percent. It might take a little bit of practice before you are successful in being responsible for your own complete awareness of a situation and paying complete attention to it. But once you get there you will find that you think with a clearer mind and are less susceptible to distractions—both internal and external!

There are several things that can prevent us from embracing mindfulness, the most common of all is being judgmental. It is easy to prejudge a situation before we are fully involved in it. This is something that is especially prevalent in the workplace. If you have a generally negative opinion of your job, and all that it involves, then you are likely going to approach the majority of your tasks during the day half-heartedly, perhaps even resentfully. Removing judgment from your mind is the best way to allow mindfulness in and bring back a sense of positivity to your work.

This In Turn will help you to stay present and therefore energized during the day.

The best way to overcome judgment is to consciously make an effort to notice when you do it, not just at work but in other areas of your life, too. Once you recognize how often you do it, and often with little to no reason, you can start to change this thought process. When you notice that you have pre-judged a situation, backtrack your thought process and try to look at it in a different way. For example, if you feel like you are being forced to do a task that you believe to be pointless, try to assess what the reasons for this task are and how it can be of benefit—both to your job on the whole and the things you might learn from it.

Sleep

Finally, and incredibly importantly, pay attention to the amount and the quality of sleep you are getting. If you are not sleeping uninterrupted for between six and eight hours a night then you are sabotaging your own energy. Adequate sleep at night is absolutely essential if you want to get through the day without wanting to head back to bed.

A common reason for failing to hit this sleep quota is the distraction of technology and communication. Switching off all of your electronic devices and having some calm, quiet time at least one hour before you go to bed will help you to avoid this problem. It can be incredibly tempting to check your messages, tweets, posts, etc., during this hour but you will soon get out of the habit and begin to look forward to the downtime that precedes bedtime.

Use the time before bed for relaxing activities such as meditation, reading, or taking a long bath. You could also designate this as family time to catch up with those closest to you.

While we sleep our body is hard at work regenerating, healing, growing, and processing nutrients from the food we have eaten during the day. Not allowing enough time for these essential processes to happen can wreak havoc within the body and will soon led to some unappealing health problems, not to mention the detriment it will have on productivity and overall wellbeing.

In order to strive for the sleep pattern your body craves then you have to treat sleep as a priority in your life. Make sure you aim to get to bed at the same time every night so that your body and mind sync with your routine. As you start to fall asleep at the same time each night, you will notice that you begin to wake at the same time each morning, too. When you do wake it will be in a refreshed state, full of the energy that your body has worked to provide you with during your sleep. If you live with other people then don't be afraid to tell them of your new bedtime routine and ensure that they respect your need for peace and quiet during this time.

In order for your sleep routine to be as successful as possible you must also address your eating habits. Trying to eat each meal at approximately the same time each day will allow your body to establish a rhythm that it can work with. Having your final meal of the day at least a few hours before you go to bed will give your digestive system enough time to do its thing—meaning you will not still be allocating energy to this process while you are trying to sleep. This in turn means that your energy can be fully focused on the regenerating, healing, growing, and nutrition processing that your body really wants to be doing!

Conclusion

Putting It All Together...

So this is it... the end. Well, of this book that is, but certainly not for the amazing you. I have given you the information and tools that I use in my every day life in the hope that you will see how easy it is to start making simple but effective changes in your life that will, in turn, give you an abundance of health, energy, and happiness. Starting with what foods to eat every single day to simple yet totally effective yoga poses, breathing exercises, meditation, and affirmations which really only need to take a few minutes out of your day if that is all you have. My advice to you is to just get them in—somehow, someway.

Many people find that change can be hard but when you have a clear ambition in mind, and the support to get there, it is well within your grasp to achieve what you want. The support I am talking about comes from the Simple Rules that I have equipped you with.

The Simple Rules are both the journey and
the end goal, they guide you to creating the
change you want in your health and wellbeing

By combining a healthy, plant-based diet, yoga, meditation, breathing, and affirmations, you are constructively making positive changes in your life with a range of tools to keep you motivated. These things all work best in conjunction with each other and you will find that as you progress in one, you progress in all.

If you are still a bit cautious about getting started then begin by writing a list of the things you want to achieve. This list can be as short or as long as you want, and the goals you list can be simple short-term things or long-term ambitions. Once you have your list, go through each item and imagine how each of the things mentioned in the Simple Rules can help you to get there. Perhaps you have written that you want to train for a marathon but you have little to no experience of running. So first of all consider your diet—how will the Simple Rules give you the body and the energy you need to persevere? Then move on to yoga and think about how improving your strength and flexibility will assist you with this goal. And on and on. I guarantee that the majority of your ambitions can be worked toward in some way by following these Simple Rules, sometimes in the most unexpected way!

It is possible to manifest the life you want by making small progressive changes both internally and externally. But remember, it has to be a total effort. You can't decide to eat well some days and then have a junk food fest the next day. Just like you can't do one yoga session and then sit on the sofa for a week in front of the TV.

Even the most pessimistic person can strip that negativity away, if they truly spend some time working to figure out what the root cause of their attitude is. If this is you, and you dedicate some time to self-analysis, you can soon move toward an optimism that will change the way you look at everything in your life.

> With the Simple Rules to keep you healthy, happy, and focused there is no limit to the self-love, self-worth, and dreams that can develop.

It is important to approach the Simple Rules with an open mind and the willingness to change.

As your attitude shifts, you will notice that so, too, does your language. You will use more positive, life-affirming words, both in your interactions with other people and subconsciously. If you find that this doesn't come naturally to you then make an effort to make it so. Surrounding yourself with positivity doesn't just apply to your environment and community, there is also a lot to be gained from using motivational language, even for the simplest of tasks. For example, instead of telling yourself that you are going to do something, try to be more present and tell yourself that you are doing it!

Most of all just believe that the life you
want is within your reach and trust that
you have the power to make it a reality.

Mindfulness will become second nature to you after you have lived by the Simple Rules for just a few months and you will discover that happiness is not as hard to find as perhaps you previously thought. You may even find as you continue along this journey that your goals change, as you become happier and more comfortable with your body, weight, relationships, and job. As we pay less attention to the external negatives and focus on ourselves, we often find that the things we thought we disliked were merely distractions preventing us from addressing the real issue.

Bonus: Happiness Habits

There are things you will start to notice about yourself as you become this new amazing you. These things are typical habits of happy people and are a sure sign that you have become more connected with yourself and your life.

1. Happy people are able to put themselves first with the added bonus of realizing that self-love is not a selfish act. This self-love in no way means that happy people have less time for other people, it simply means that they are caring for themselves in the way that they should.

2. Happy people are better prepared to accept the temporary nature of certain things. Nothing was meant to last forever and deep-down inside we all know this. Having trouble letting go of a job or a relationship is natural, but true happiness brings about the ability to appreciate what was and understand that it is no more.

3. Happy people don't care how others perceive them. They know who they are and what makes them great. They don't need the validation of others and this is an incredibly liberating feeling. Similarly, they are able to not take rejection personally as they understand that this means something was simply not meant to be. By accepting a rejection instead of dwelling on it, happy people have much more time and energy to put toward continued positivity.

So, as you work toward building the new, healthier you, rest assured that you will find your happiness and become the amazing new you that you wanted to be and in fact, always were. And don't forget to share your positivity with others in your life. Be generous. Be kind and be willing to share your experience in order to help those you love re-discover themselves too. Being the best version of yourself is actually really simple.

Namaste.

References

Introduction

1. Yokoyama, Y. "Vegetarian Diets and Blood Pressure," *JAMA Internal Medicine*, February 24, 2014 [Epub ahead of print]
2. http://www.livescience.com/43627-vegetarian-diets-lower-blood-pressure.html; accessed 10/10/2015
3. http://www.cancer.gov/about-cancer/causes-prevention/risk/diet/antioxidants-fact-sheet#q3-; accessed 10/10/2015

Chapter 1: Eat One Green Leafy Veg Every Day

1. https://www.pcrm.org/health/cancer-resources/diet-cancer/nutrition/how-carotenoids-help-protect-against-cancer; accessed 10/10/2015
2. http://health.howstuffworks.com/wellness/food-nutrition/vitamin-supplements/what-are-carotenoids.htm; accessed 10/10/2015
3. *ibid*
4. http://www.healwithfood.org/skincancer/diet.php; accessed 10/10/2015
5. http://www3.amherst.edu/~dmirwin/Reports/NCIFactSheet.htm; accessed 10/10/2015

6. http://www.cancer.gov/about-cancer/causes-prevention/risk/diet/cruciferous-vegetables-fact-sheet#q3; accessed 10/10/2015

7. http://cebp.aacrjournals.org/content/8/5/447.full; accessed 10/10/2015

8. http://www.todaysdietitian.com/newarchives/100111p20.shtml; accessed 10/10/2015

9. http://www.ncbi.nlm.nih.gov/pmc/articles/PMC2737735; accessed 10/10/2015

10. http://lpi.oregonstate.edu/mic/food-beverages/cruciferous-vegetables; accessed 10/10/2015

11. http://www.naturalhealth365.com/cancer_treatments/glucosinolates.html; accessed 10/10/2015

12. http://blog.lifeextension.com/2013/03/vegetables-support-gut-immunity.html; accessed 10/10/2015

13. *ibid*

14. http://articles.mercola.com/sites/articles/archive/2015/07/16/link-between-processed-food-depression.aspx; accessed 10/10/2015

15. http://www.mentalhealth.org.uk/content/assets/pdf/publications/healthy_eating_depression.pdf; accessed 10/10/2015

16. http://americanpregnancy.org/pregnancy-health/folic-acid/

17. http://www.whfoods.com/genpage.php?tname=foodspice&dbid=43; accessed 10/10/2015

18. http://www.cancer.gov/about-cancer/causes-prevention/risk/diet/cruciferous-vegetables-fact-sheet; accessed 10/27/2015

19. http://www.sciencedaily.com/releases/2015/05/150515134827.htm; accessed 02/11/2015

20. http://www.medicaldaily.com/mental-health-benefits-probiotics-good-bacteria-may-improve-mood-fight-depression-328882; accessed 10/27/2015

Chapter 2: Get Heart Healthy with Whole Grains

1. http://health.howstuffworks.com/diseases-conditions/cardiovascular/cholesterol/foods-that-lower-cholesterol2.htm; accessed 10/12/2015

2. http://www.heart.org/HEARTORG/GettingHealthy/NutritionCenter/HealthyDietGoals/Whole-Grains-and-Fiber_UCM_303249_Article.jsp; accessed 10/12/2015

3. Hollaender, P. *et al*, "Whole-grain and blood lipid changes in apparently healthy adults: a systematic review and meta-analysis of randomized controlled studies," *American Journal of Clinical Nutrition*, August 2015 [Epub ahead of print]

4. Caselato-Sousa, V. *et al*. "Intake of heat-expanded amaranth grain reverses endothelial dysfunction in hypercholesterolemic rabbits," *Food & Function*, November 2014; 5(12): 3281–6

5. Postgraduate Medical School, University of Surrey, "Short-term effects of whole-grain wheat on appetite and food intake in healthy adults: a pilot study," *British Journal of Nutrition*, April 2011; 1–4 [Epub ahead of print]

6. Kazemzadeh, M. *et al*. "Effect of Brown Rice Consumption on Inflammatory Marker and Cardiovascular Risk Factors among Overweight and Obese Non-menopausal Female Adults," *International Journal of Preventive Medicine*, April 2012; 5(4): 478–88

7. Satya, S. *et al*. "Putting the Whole Grain Puzzle Together: Health Benefits Associated with Whole Grains," *British Journal of Nutrition*, Apr 2011: 1–4 [Epub ahead of print]

8. Kazemzadeh, M. *et al*. "Effect of Brown Rice Consumption on Inflammatory Marker and Cardiovascular Risk Factors among Overweight and Obese Non-menopausal Female Adults," *International Journal of Preventive Medicine*, April 2014; 5(4): 478–88

9. http://www.cdc.gov/bloodpressure/facts.htm; accessed 10/12/2015

10. Kristensen, M. *et al*. "Whole grain compared with refined wheat decreases the percentage of body fat following a 12-week, energy-restricted dietary intervention in postmenopausal women," *The Journal of Nutrition*, April 2012; 142(4): 710–6

11. Andersson, U. *et al.* "Metabolic effects of whole grain wheat and whole grain rye in the C57BL/6J mouse," *Nutrition,* February 2010; 26(2): 230–9; Epub July 31, 2009

12. InterAct Consortium, "More Evidence That a High-Fiber Diet May Prevent Type 2 Diabetes," *Diabetologia,* May 2015 [Epub ahead of print]

13. Huang, T. *et al.* "Consumption of whole grains and cereal fiber and total and cause-specific mortality: prospective analysis of 367,442 individuals," *BMC Medicine,* Mar 4 2015; 13: 59

14. Williams, P. *et al.* "The benefits of breakfast cereal consumption: a systematic review of the evidence base," *Advances in Nutrition,* Sep 15 2014; 5(5): 636S–73S

15. Sun, Q. *et al.* "White rice, brown rice, and risk of type 2 diabetes in US men and women," *Archives of Internal Medicine,* June 2010; 170(11): 96–9

16. http://www.medicalnewstoday.com/articles/287049.php; accessed 10/12/2015

17. http://www.cliffordawright.com/caw/food/entries/display.php/topic_id/9/id/122/; accessed 10/12/2015

Chapter 3: Out with Refined Sugars, In with Natural Sweeteners

1. http://www.usda.gov/factbook/chapter2.pdf; accessed 10/12/2015

2. http://bamboocorefitness.com/not-so-sweet-the-average-american-consumes-150-170-pounds-of-sugar-each-year/; accessed 10/12/2015

3. http://advances.nutrition.org/content/4/2/220.full; accessed 10/12/2015

4. http://www.ncbi.nlm.nih.gov/pubmed/23719144; accessed 10/12/2015

5. http://www.builtlean.com/2014/01/23/coke-10-teaspoons-sugar; accessed 02/11/2015

6. http://www.livestrong.com/article/306908-how-many-calories-does-soda-have; accessed 02/11/2015

7. http://paleoleap.com/10-reasons-why-fructose-is-bad/; accessed 10/12/2015

8. http://authoritynutrition.com/why-is-fructose-bad-for-you/; accessed 10/12/2015

9. http://ajcn.nutrition.org/content/86/4/895.ful; accessed 10/12/2015

10. http://www.health.harvard.edu/heart-health/abundance-of-fructose-not-good-for-the-liver-heart; accessed 10/12/2015

11. http://www.ncbi.nlm.nih.gov/pmc/articles/PMC2235907/; accessed 10/12/2015

12. http://www.ncbi.nlm.nih.gov/pubmed/19817641; accessed 10/12/2015

13. http://www.ncbi.nlm.nih.gov/pubmed/22888839; accessed 10/12/2015

14. http://www.aicr.org/cancer-research-update/2012/december_5_2012/cru-flavonoids-prevention.html; accessed 10/12/2015

15. http://articles.mercola.com/sites/articles/archive/2011/05/27/can-eating-local-honey-cure-allergies.aspx; accessed 10/12/2015

16. http://www.scientificamerican.com/article/honey-heightens-athletic/; accessed 10/13/2015

17. http://www.diabetes.org/food-and-fitness/food/what-can-i-eat/making-healthy-food-choices/coconut-palm-sugar.html; accessed 10/12/2015

Chapter 4: Goodbye Refined Oils, Hello Healthy Unrefined Oils

1. http://www.ncbi.nlm.nih.gov/pmc/articles/PMC2802050/; accessed 10/12/2015

2. http://customers.hbci.com/~wenonah/new/canola.htm; accessed 10/12/2015

3. http://vanessaruns.com/2011/02/08/gmos-and-why-you-should-never-use-canola-oil/; accessed 10/13/2015

4. http://bebrainfit.com/coconut-oil-benefits-brain/; accessed 10/13/2015

5. http://healthimpactnews.com/2012/coconut-oil-and-alzheimers-disease-the-news-is-spreading/; accessed 10/13/2015

6. http://authoritynutrition.com/extra-virgin-olive-oil/; accessed 10/13/2015

7. http://www.betterhealth.vic.gov.au/bhcv2/bhcarticles.nsf/pages/olive_oil?open; accessed 10/13/2015

8. http://www.oliveoiltimes.com/olive-oil-health-benefits; accessed 10/13/2015

9. http://www.nhs.uk/news/2013/02February/Pages/Mediterranean-diet-cuts-heart-disease-and-stroke-risk.aspx; accessed 10/13/2015

10. http://www.whfoods.com/genpage.php?tname=news&dbid=3; accessed 10/13/2015

11. http://www.livestrong.com/article/408569-the-effects-of-flaxseed-oil-on-blood-pressure/; accessed 10/13/2015

12. http://whfoods.org/genpage.php?tname=foodspice&dbid=81; accessed 10/13/2015

13. http://www.spiritofhealthkc.com/portfolio/gallstones-natural-healing-protocol/; accessed 10/13/2015

14. http://www.herbwisdom.com/herb-flaxseed-oil.html; accessed 10/13/2015

Chapter 5: Get the Fat on Good Fats

1. http://www.neurobiologyofaging.org/article/S0197-4580(14)00355-8/abstract?cc=y=; accessed 10/13/2015

2. http://www.tfx.org.uk/page131.html; accessed 10/13/2015

3. http://journals.cambridge.org/download.php?file=%2FNRR%2FNRR21_02%2FS0954422408110964a.pdf&code=2d0706bd7e41929c1e3a1a9fe14560df; accessed 10/13/2015

4. http://www.webmd.com/infertility-and-reproduction/news/20070112/trans-fats-infertility; accessed 10/13/2015

References
₋₋₋₋₋₋₋₋₋₋₋₋

5. http://www.dietdoctor.com/saturated-fat-completely-safe-according-new-big-review-science; accessed 10/13/2015

6. http://www.diabetes.org/food-and-fitness/food/what-can-i-eat/making-healthy-food-choices/fats-and-diabetes.html; accessed 10/13/2015

7. http://www.ncbi.nlm.nih.gov/pmc/articles/PMC2654180/; accessed 10/13/2015

8. http://greatist.com/eat/healthy-fats-best-foods-for-brain-health; accessed 10/13/2015

9. http://www.healthambition.com/using-almonds-for-weight-loss/; accessed 10/13/2015

10. http://www.healthline.com/health/diabetes/almonds; accessed 10/13/2015

11. http://www.doctoroz.com/article/brain-diet; accessed 10/13/2015

12. http://www.everydayhealth.com/diabetes-pictures/new-diabetes-superfoods-you-should-try.aspx; accessed 10/13/2015

13. http://www.naturalnews.com/037568_pumpkins_blood_glucose_enlarged_prostate.html; accessed 10/13/2015

14. http://woman.thenest.com/foods-high-phytoestrogens-2327.html; accessed 10/13/2015

15. https://www.endocrine.org/news-room/press-release-archives/2002/20020419; accessed 10/13/2015

16. http://www.livestrong.com/article/517596-pumpkin-seeds-blood-pressure/; accessed 10/13/2015

17. http://whfoods.org/genpage.php?tname=foodspice&dbid=81; accessed 10/13/2015

18. http://www.naturalnews.com/023744_flax_oil.html; accessed 10/13/2015

19. http://articles.mercola.com/sites/articles/archive/2001/07/21/flaxseed-part-two.aspx; accessed 10/13/2015

20. https://www.drfuhrman.com/library/cancer_flax.aspx; accessed 10/13/2015

Chapter 6: Get the Super Back into Your Diet

1. http://www.health.com/health/gallery/0,,20430736,00.html; accessed 10/13/2015

2. http://www.canceractive.com/cancer-active-page-link.aspx?n=531; accessed 10/13/2015

3. http://www.mesothelioma.com/blog/authors/jackie/5-superfoods-for-cancer-patients.htm; accessed 10/13/2015

4. http://www.nhs.uk/livewell/superfoods/pages/what-are-superfoods.aspx; accessed 10/13/2015

5. http://www.livestrong.com/article/236254-top-10-super-foods-for-antioxidants/; accessed 10/13/2015

6. http://www.medicalnewstoday.com/articles/282929.php; accessed 10/13/2015

7. https://www.bhf.org.uk/heart-health/preventing-heart-disease/healthy-eating; accessed 10/13/2015

8. http://www.livestrong.com/article/370124-how-to-dilate-blood-vessels-with-herbs/; accessed 10/13/2015

9. http://www.ehow.co.uk/way_5595589_foods-eat-blood-vessels-dilate.html; accessed 10/13/2015

10. http://www.webmd.com/healthy-aging/features/anti-aging-diet; accessed 10/13/2015

11. http://www.ncbi.nlm.nih.gov/books/NBK92756/; accessed 10/13/2015

12. http://articles.mercola.com/sites/articles/archive/2011/07/01/spirulina-the-amazing-super-food-youve-never-heard-of.aspxl accessed 10/13/2015

13. http://articles.mercola.com/sites/articles/archive/2011/07/01/spirulina-the-amazing-super-food-youve-never-heard-of.aspx; accessed 10/13/2015

14. http://www.webmd.com/food-recipes/protein; accessed 10/13/2015

15. http://www.bee-pollen-benefits.com; accessed 10/13/2015

16. http://www.hindawi.com/journals/ecam/2015/297425/; accessed 10/13/2015

17. http://www.mercola.com/article/diet/bee_pollen.htm; accessed 10/13/2015

18. http://www.webmd.com/vitamins-supplements/ingredientmono-78-bee%20pollen.aspx?activeingredientid=78&activeingredientname=bee%20pollen; accessed 10/13/2015

19. http://www.vanderbilt.edu/AnS/psychology/health_psychology/beepollen.htm; accessed 10/13/2015

20. http://dailysuperfoodlove.com/2852/21-fantastic-benefits-of-cacao/; accessed 10/13/2015

21. http://www.naturalnews.com/041916_cacao_scientific_research_health_benefits.htm;accessed 10/13/2015]

Chapter 7: Five Simple Rules on Eating Out

1. http://www.livestrong.com/article/528064-does-eating-apples-before-meals-help-you-lose-weight/; accessed 10/14/2015

2. http://www.webmd.com/dict/fiber-weight-control; accessed 10/14/2015

3. http://www.mayoclinic.org/diseases-conditions/heart-disease/in-depth/red-wine/art-20048281; accessed 10/14/2015

4. http://www.heartmdinstitute.com/video-library/web-shows/myth-buster-series/437-is-red-wine-and-alcohol-good-for-your-heart; accessed 10/14/2015

Chapter 8: Channel Your Superhero Powers

1. http://www.ncbi.nlm.nih.gov/pubmed/16353426; accessed 10/14/2015

2. http://www.livestrong.com/article/182548-how-to-get-rid-of-cortisol-fat/;accessed 10/14/2015

3. http://www.wholeliving.com/208200/curb-cravings-yoga; accessed 10/14/2015

4. http://www.yogajournal.com/meditation/mindful-eating-meditation-manage-food-cravings/; accessed 10/14/2015

Chapter 9: Easy Tips to Keep You Going...

1. http://www.theguardian.com/lifeandstyle/2015/jun/01/office-workers-on-feet-standing-fours-hours-day-study-health; accessed 10/14/2015

2. http://www.washingtonpost.com/news/wonkblog/wp/2015/06/02/medical-researchers-have-figured-out-how-much-time-is-okay-to-spend-sitting-each-day/; accessed 10/14/2015

3. http://www.health.harvard.edu/blog/much-sitting-linked-heart-disease-diabetes-premature-death-201501227618; accessed 10/14/2015

4. http://www.nhs.uk/livewell/fitness/pages/sitting-and-sedentary-behaviour-are-bad-for-your-health.aspx; accessed 10/14/2015

Index

ABOUT THE AUTHOR

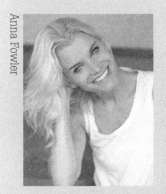

Anna Fowler

Julie Montagu is one of London's top yoga and nutrition teachers. As Cosmopolitan said: *"...the name Julie Montagu is talked about with the sort of reverence reserved for the Dalai Lama. (Her Sunday yoga class gets so packed that she often teaches standing on a radiator. True Story.)"*

Julie stars in the TV show *Ladies of London* (US Bravo and ITVBe), is the brains behind her online courses at The Flexi Foodie Academy, and has created her own superfood energy snacks, JUB. Julie's workshops on Self-Love, Letting Go and Happiness have been sell-out successes. She lives in London with her husband and four children.

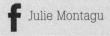 Julie Montagu   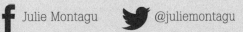 @juliemontagu   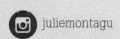 juliemontagu

www.juliemontagu.com
www.theflexifoodie.com
www.jubfood.com

We hope you enjoyed this Hay House book. If you'd like to receive our online catalog featuring additional information on Hay House books and products, or if you'd like to find out more about the Hay Foundation, please contact:

Hay House, Inc., P.O. Box 5100, Carlsbad, CA 92018-5100
(760) 431-7695 or (800) 654-5126
(760) 431-6948 (fax) or (800) 650-5115 (fax)
www.hayhouse.com® • www.hayfoundation.org

Published and distributed in Australia by:
Hay House Australia Pty. Ltd., 18/36 Ralph St., Alexandria NSW 2015
Phone: 612-9669-4299 • *Fax:* 612-9669-4144 • www.hayhouse.com.au

Published and distributed in the United Kingdom by:
Hay House UK, Ltd., Astley House, 33 Notting Hill Gate, London W11 3JQ
Phone: 44-20-3675-2450 • *Fax:* 44-20-3675-2451 • www.hayhouse.co.uk

Published and distributed in the Republic of South Africa by:
Hay House SA (Pty), Ltd., P.O. Box 990, Witkoppen 2068
info@hayhouse.co.za • www.hayhouse.co.za

Published in India by: Hay House Publishers India,
Muskaan Complex, Plot No. 3, B-2, Vasant Kunj, New Delhi 110 070
Phone: 91-11-4176-1620 • *Fax:* 91-11-4176-1630 • www.hayhouse.co.in

Distributed in Canada by: Raincoast Books,
2440 Viking Way, Richmond, B.C. V6V 1N2
Phone: 1-800-663-5714 • *Fax:* 1-800-565-3770 • www.raincoast.com

---

Take Your Soul on a Vacation

Visit www.HealYourLife.com® to regroup, recharge,
and reconnect with your own magnificence.
Featuring blogs, mind-body-spirit news, and
life-changing wisdom from Louise Hay and friends.

Visit www.HealYourLife.com today!